Brian Ford is Chairman
at the Institute of Biolog,
meeting on the history of BSE in 1990. He has presented many programmes on radio and TV, including *Food for Thought* for Channel 4 and *Where Are You Taking Us?* for the BBC. Among the 70 editions of his books published around the world are *The Food Book*, and his much-acclaimed textbook *Microbiology and Food*. Brian Ford, who is the science editor of *The Guinness Book of Records*, lives in Cambridgeshire.

BSE: THE FACTS

Mad Cow Disease and the Risk to Mankind

Brian J. Ford

Sector Chairman, Institute of Biology

CORGI BOOKS

BSE: THE FACTS
A CORGI BOOK : 0 552 14530 0

First publication in Great Britain

PRINTING HISTORY
Corgi edition published 1996

Corgi Books are published by Transworld Publishers Ltd,
61–63 Uxbridge Road, Ealing, London W5 5SA,
in Australia by Transworld Publishers (Australia) Pty Ltd,
15–25 Helles Avenue, Moorebank, NSW 2170,
and in New Zealand by Transworld Publishers (NZ) Ltd,
3 William Pickering Drive, Albany, Auckland.

Set in 10/12pt Sabon by
Phoenix Typesetting, Ilkley, West Yorkshire

Reproduced, printed and bound in Great Britain by
Cox & Wyman Ltd, Reading, Berks.

CONTENTS

PREFACE

The terrible tragedy of mad cow disease has touched everyone in Britain. Yet there has been no source of background information. The few books on the subject are either specialist publications, and are naturally somewhat terse and esoteric, or they seem to set out to be frightening. There must be people who would like something different. Perhaps this summary of the facts, from a personal standpoint, will satisfy some of them.

Over the years I have discussed the research with countless biologist colleagues, and could not recall them all. I have learned much from Ray Bradley, formerly of the Central Veterinary Laboratory, Chris Bostock of the Institute for Animal Health, and R. C. Lowson of the Ministry of Agriculture, Fisheries and Food. They all lectured at the BSE meeting I organized in 1990, and provided so very much food for thought. I have had the chance to exchange personal views from all sides of the controversy with John Pattison, Michael Young, Stephen Dealler and Richard Lacey. Some friends on the Internet have sent in valuable information, and my warmest thanks to them, too. They'll know who they are.

Much of the detailed information in this book derives from the research of some of the greatest scientific minds of our time, and some of them are cited in the text. The unravelling events of April 1996 were recorded with great skill by journalists to whose accounts I owe so much. Britain boasts some of the finest science correspondents and political writers, and I am particularly indebted to Robin McKie, Jonathan Calvert, Dean Nelson, Steve Connor, Roger Highfield, David Brown, Nigel Hawkes, Victoria MacDonald, Mark Watts, Boris Johnson, Adrian Berry, Charles Reiss, John Craig, Richard Palmer, and Peter Martin for their tireless efforts and literary skill. Among the journals I have consulted most frequently are *Proceedings of the Royal Society, Nature,* the *Lancet* and *The Economist.*

As this extended essay was taking shape I received some vital insights from some of the wisest scientists I know, and, if they don't mind too much, would like to mention Peter Biggs, former President of the Institute of Biology, John Slade the virologist, and Brian Heap, the Institute of Biology's current President. If I have failed to learn the lessons of your wisdom, blame the pupil. It was not the fault of the teachers.

1

TAKE A CHANCE AND LIVE

The spring of 1996 was the latest anyone could remember. There is a peach tree in Cambridge which normally blooms in February. Its blossoms stayed closed until the last week of April. By this late date grass growth had struggled to reach three inches, and beef cattle were being turned out to graze for the first time since winter.

For a month, a new scourge had been feared across the land. Over a dozen young Europeans were dead, their brains destroyed by a horrifying disease never before seen in the West. The British government was launching a unique case against Brussels in the courts, and the cattle industry was facing ruin. Farmers had been offered less than £500 per head for animals due to be culled. On 16 April the Government had made their final offer:

- £550 million to slaughter cattle over 30 months
- £118 million support to the carcase-rendering industry
- A total of £240 million for abattoirs, farmers with bull calves on their hands, and farms raising beef.

It was politicians such as the Agriculture Minister Douglas Hogg who claimed the limelight, but it was

Brussels who called the tune. British attitudes were based on politics, rather than science. The National Farmers Union President, Sir David Naish, was in No. 10 Downing Street so often he was mistaken for a politician more than once.

Little was heard of other crucial topics. What about the tragic plight of families, mourning their young dead? How much of the problem was caused by government in the first place? And what was the truth of the matter? Behind all the activity designed to boost public confidence, was beef safe to eat, or not? Why were British consumers allowed to eat as much beef as they liked, whilst the same meat was considered too dangerous for other Europeans? Were the British expendable, or were there deeper forces at work?

Before we unravel the story, let's set the risks in proportion. How did you come by this book? If you drove to the bookshop, you had a chance a thousand times greater of being seriously injured or killed than those tragic young people had of dying from eating beef. Are you reading it on a train? You are ten times as likely to be killed in a railway accident within a year.

New risks are regularly reported. On 21 April 1996 the *Sunday Times* said that scrapie was spread by ticks. On 23 April, the Government launched a counter-offensive at Luxembourg, although it was their action which had caused many of the problems. Stephen Dealler, in his colloquial account released on 24 April 1996, lengthily recounted official attempts to hinder his enquiries.

There is much we must learn from this disastrous outbreak. The British government has played with our fate, censoring news and laundering the facts in order to safeguard their own priorities. We have all been exposed to risks from which we should have been protected. But we all take risks whatever we do, and most of them we ought to avoid. There are cancer-causing chemicals in cress and kippers, and the risk of death lurks in a can of lager beer. Living means we die, and our concern must not be allowed to transmute into unreasonable fear.

The Hazards of Eating

Eating is a risky business. It always has been. You might choke on an olive, contract cancer from celery or a coronary from cake. Eat too much and you are threatened with obesity; too little and there could be a risk from anorexia. Human history has been marked by food scares, by fashionable beliefs about the diet. The news about beef is only the latest in a long line of panics.

If there is anyone in a worse situation than a beef-eater at the moment, it is a scientist. I am always being asked: 'Why did nobody give any hint that this might happen?' They did. The pronouncements of biologists have been misquoted by the authorities. All the reports which I have read examine this fascinating subject objectively and honestly. It is the official spokesmen who have singled out the phrases that suited them and quoted them out of context. For all our scientific knowledge, in this most technological era in history, the public are kept at arm's length from what really goes on. Government is unable to handle scientific facts and figures. The comments that leak out to the press are misleading.

The BSE episode has been shamefully mismanaged. It still is. Some of the principal research workers, people of integrity and experience, have been ordered not to speak to anyone about their work, nor to reveal their own opinions. There has been deliberate misrepresentation of the facts by the Government. We are moving into a highly scientific age, yet few in government understand what is involved.

The public have become increasingly disenfranchised

from science, and we are heading into an era where they cannot challenge what they are being told. Modern science lacks the broad-minded, interdisciplinary approach it needs to tackle new problems like this. This is an exceedingly dangerous situation, and the sad saga of BSE could forewarn us of the need to address new problems in the future. Yesterday's conventions are not enough for the challenge of tomorrow.

BSE – the Problem

There are several factors which make this outbreak unusual.

- First, its nature. This is not just an illness which goes away or gets better. In this dreadful disease, the mind collapses. Tiny holes appear scattered through the brain tissue. There is something peculiarly threatening about an attack on the brain.
- Secondly, there is the outcome. Every case is fatal. There have never been any recoveries. Death from the illness is always certain.
- Third is its insidiousness. This is a disease which may be passed on through doing what most people have done for thousands of years – eating beef. It doesn't come from poor hygiene or carelessness, as food poisoning can.
- Fourth is the mysterious origin. This is a fascinating condition. There is no microbe as the cause. There isn't a virus for cow disease. The public has been watching the unravelling of the structure of DNA reported from laboratories around the world. Every known form of infection has always had DNA (or RNA, its 'messenger') at its heart. But these new diseases don't even seem to have that. This is a completely novel form of infective agent. Nobody understands how it works.
- Then there is the factor of the advice people have been given. In specialist subjects the public like to take the best advice avail-

able. The Government have insisted for ten years that there is no risk to humans. We have to heed the advice of scientists, they said. In science we knew there was no evidence of transmission to people. There still isn't any evidence that BSE from cows can cause CJD in humans – but many words of warning were given.

- The sixth major dimension of this historic episode is the sense of fear in the public. People do not know where to go, where to turn, whom to consult. Public information has been badly handled. The information that has been released is misleading, and the facts have been concealed.

What Killed the Cannibals?

The newspapers have been filled with comment, bursting with reports as events unfold. Hundreds of outbreaks have now been reported in Switzerland. Across the United States (where a similar disease has long existed in deer) there is a desperate coast-to-coast search for infected cattle. French farmers are said to be secretly disposing of BSE-positive animals, anxious to stifle adverse comments.

What people have demanded are the facts – yet the full facts have not been available. In this book I set out the current state of knowledge, with analysis of the present extent of scientific uncertainty. Where there are areas of ignorance I try to spell them out, and where there have been examples of incompetence or muddle-headedness I will explain those, too, as far as I can.

Medical reports insist we are witnessing an outbreak of a new strain of Creutzfeldt-Jakob disease, CJD. That is not what the microscope reveals. Within the brains of these young people are not the signs of CJD, but those of a more dramatic affliction by far. The appearance is that of kuru, the 'laughing death' of Papua New Guinea.

The cannibals' plague has been recreated in the West.

Laying down the Law

Governments like to assume that there are hard and fast rules you can impose on the public. That's how all governments operate – they exist only to lay down the rules. In matters of personal choice, no two people are ever exactly the same. Individuals need to make up their own minds, and form opinions based on the essential facts of the matter. We regularly do things that are insanely dangerous, like smoke a cigarette or drive round a corner at speed. The chances of dying from eating beef are, on present evidence, hundreds of times less than those of driving to the store to buy it.

The subject is also filled with half-digested facts. Official spokesmen keep talking about food entering the human 'food chain'. This is a fundamental misunderstanding. In a food *chain*, some food is eaten by an animal, which is in turn eaten by something else, which falls prey to something larger . . . and so on. A worm contaminated by insecticides passes them up through a 'food chain' to other organisms, which concentrate them further. The predator at the end of the line – a bird of prey – contains so much of the poison that it can't lay sound eggs.

Infected food is only entering the human 'food chain' if it – or we – are being eaten by some other species. The infected food is not part of our food 'chain' at all, but part of our food *supply*. The meat is in our diet. Politicians and others who don't understand nutrition like to use the term 'food chain' because it sounds technical and might impress their listeners. Don't fall for it. Anyone using that term doesn't know their amino-acids from their elbow.

Coming to Terms with Risk

Little attempt has been made to think these matters through to a sensible conclusion. For instance, some British suppliers now proudly boast that they use only imported beef. Much of this is tainted with hormones and antibiotics (used illegally in many foreign countries). Some of the meat now being imported is of a far lower standard of safety than the domestic product which has been rejected.

We are equally bad at understanding risks in our daily lives, and government regulations do not always fit reality. 'Everyone must drive on the same side of the road!' says a government edict, and nobody will argue with the sense of that. But with health matters it is never so simple. 'Smoking kills!' say government health warnings, as George Burns puffs away at his pre-breakfast cigar on the morning of his 100th birthday.

The muddled thinking about the safety of beef was summed up by a Danish woman glimpsed in a TV report at the height of the initial panic. Was she frightened of beef? 'Oh yes,' she said. 'Since the first reports I do not eat any beef, not English beef, not even Danish beef. The risks may be small, but they frighten me.' She paused and, to calm her fears, raised her right hand. It carried a cigarette. She took a long draw, pulling the smoke deep into her lungs.

'Eating beef,' she announced, 'is a risk.'

Then she blew out the cigarette smoke, rich in cancer-causing chemicals, dense with tiny particles that damage the lungs, and sparkling with iridescent droplets of toxic tar.

'Beef is too big a chance for me, at any rate,' she said, and coughed, softly.

And I'll bet she drove home.

2

MAD COWS AND ENGLISHMEN

The market town of Ashford, in Kent, lies in rolling countryside at the heart of the 'garden of England'. For generations of Londoners, it was at the centre of the hop-picking trips which provided working holidays for the impecunious families who came to help bring in the harvest. It now boasts a major international rail station which funnels train traffic through the tunnel to France. Ashford typifies the British way of life, both ancient and modern.

Over Easter 1985 a local veterinary surgeon, Colin Whitaker, was called to a farm to see a cow which was unwell. She was behaving oddly, moving unsteadily on shaky legs. Her mood had changed. Normally docile and compliant, she was becoming hyperactive, and aggressive towards the farmer. In some ways the disease looked like the staggers, a condition which has been known for centuries. The staggers results from a lack of magnesium in the diet, and it can be cured by treatment with supplements. Magnesium did nothing for this poor beast, and Mr Whitaker soon realized he was witnessing something he had never seen before. It looked like the long-known disease of sheep we call scrapie – but infecting a cow.

The case was brought to the attention of the Central Veterinary Laboratory in Weybridge, Surrey. One of their pathologists, Dr G. A. H. Wells, concluded that this was a previously unrecorded condition. By November 1986 it had acquired the name it bears to this day – bovine spongiform encephalopathy, or BSE for short. The first presentation on the subject was a lecture to the British Veterinary Association in July 1987.

A Decade of Study

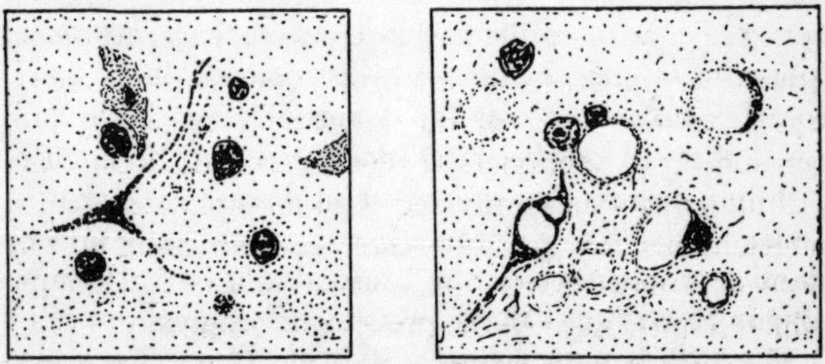

Fig 1: Normal and Spongy brain sections

In a section of normal brain tissue (left), *cells are evenly scattered and a smooth matrix between the cells holds them in position. In spongiform disease* (right) *abnormal proteins force the nerve cells to form conspicuous holes, or vacuoles. The brain cannot function normally in this state.*

For about ten years this new and fascinating disease has lurked around the corridors of science. It is a strange condition in which the brain changes its structure. The normal communities of brain cells, connected together in a vast array like a trillion telephone exchanges, break down. The smooth systems of proteins of which the brain is composed start to grow at odd angles, and small gaps appear inside the nerve cells. The brain loses power. Billions of the tiny signals which move between the brain cells start to go wrong. Some are sent to incorrect places. Others stop dead in their tracks. Under the microscope, the damage to the brain makes the tissues appear much like a sponge, and this is where the disease acquired its complicated-looking identity.

Bovine spongiform encephalopathy is not such a strange name as it seems. The brain, in Greek, is the *enkephalon*, so a pathological condition of the brain is an encephalopathy. In these diseases the brain changes to look like a sponge, so they were dubbed spongiform encephalopathies. The newly discovered version occurred in bovine animals (like cows) so the term *bovine spongiform encephalopathy* was coined. It is only complex because it uses the quaint blend of Latin and Greek that has long been traditional in science. In English it simply means 'cow spongy-brain disease', and that is understandable to everyone. If you cannot fully understand a problem in science, translating it into a foreign tongue always gives the impression of progress.

The most famous victim of BSE was Daisy. She was a black and white Friesian suckler cow aged six years. The Friesians are the most common milk cows in Britain. Daisy is the unfortunate beast who falls about so dramatically in the early video of mad cow disease which regularly replays on TV. Her uncoordinated gait and poor bodily condition were reflected in an agitated and nervous manner. She frequently tried to rub her head, either with a front hoof, or against a wall; and soon lost the ability to walk. The videotape provides a graphic illustration of the terrible consequences of contracting spongy-brain disease. Since BSE was recognized, no cow is normally permitted to become so ill with the disease.

The youngest animal ever to contract BSE was aged

twenty months, the oldest eighteen years. However, we believe that the disease has a normal incubation period that seems to range between two-and-a-half and ten years. Its origin has been related to the feeding of untreated meat and bone-meal to cattle. Although it is not known for sure, this seems to be the most likely source of the original outbreak of BSE. Let us see why this is widely believed.

Possible Causes

At first, nobody had any idea what might have caused the illness. What were the possibilities? The full list of rival theories is explained in Chapter 14, but these were the initial targets of interest:

- Imported animals
- Imported foodstuffs
- Vaccines
- Viruses
- Pharmaceuticals, including hormones
- Agricultural chemicals, such as pesticides
- Scrapie, from contact with sheep

In a situation like this we have to look for factors common to all cases. In this way, several of the possible causes were eliminated. For example, one possibility was that the disease resulted from the powerful chemical treatments used to control pests in farm animals. Strong insecticides are used in sheep dips, and have been shown to pose a possible risk to farm-workers who are not properly protected. A theory about BSE was that it was a reaction to the insecticides used to treat warble fly in cattle. This does not seem to stand up to scrutiny, because the occurrence of BSE does not match the extent of use of the chemical treatments. There is BSE in places where the insecticides aren't used.

One single factor linking the cows with BSE was meat and bone-meal. This is the lumpy compound fed to cattle to encourage them to grow and to produce plenty of milk. It lasts well in winter storage, and it does not go off too quickly, so it is an ideal staple food for intensively reared cows. The meal can be produced in different shapes and sizes known from their shape as pencils, nuts or pellets. Farm-workers sometimes nibble at them, and it is the eating of animal feed by humans that has been proposed as a reason why some dairy farmers have contracted spongy-brain disease.

The animal feed is no longer transported in sacks or bags, but by bulk tanker. Tons of the feed is blasted under pressure up a large delivery pipe into a storage loft. The dust is pervasive, the noise unendurable (the drivers wear ear-protectors against the piercing sound of the pump). Workers inhale the dust, and if there were to be a batch of feed contaminated by an infectious bacterium there is nothing to stop an outbreak. This is another reason why all animal feed should be free of disease germs.

Many beef farms raise cattle on a diet which the farmers produce themselves. The cattle consume hay or grass, beet tops, or silage made from the farmer's own harvest of crops like maize. It was noted that many cattle reared on a diet of vegetation had not developed BSE. The cattle at risk seemed to have meat and bone-meal as the common factor. You could, of course, raise an immediate query. It was much the same as the objection to the theories about insecticides and chemical sprays – namely, why were the cattle getting ill at this particular time? The meal had been around for years, whereas BSE was suddenly spreading all over the country.

Though it is true that the meal had long been in use, the way it was made had changed. In the 1970s, meat and bone-meal was made from carcases unusable for other purposes. Unsaleable sheep carcases were among the sources used to make the meal. The carcases were heat-treated (which served to sterilize them). The ground-up remains were also treated with solvents to dissolve out the fat. At the time, fat was a valuable by-product of the industry. Since about 1980 it has not been worth recovering.

Market Forces or Greed?

During the 1980s, the farming business came under heavy pressure from what were called 'market forces'. This is often a misnomer. The market is where we buy goods and services, and market forces are the principles which maintain that supply. If a product is dangerous, or a service proves unreliable, then the market collapses. In the modern era, people do not stop to consider the market so much as their quick profit. If you can sell something cheaper at a higher price, then you can cream off the takings. If the company collapses, no matter; turn your back on the mess and start another one.

The aim of the food industry used to be quality, reliability and service. In the modern era, profit matters above all, and you can see the results all around you. Food poisoning is steadily on the increase. Substances known to make some people ill (salt, saturated fats, gluten, etc.) are marketed for short-term gain. Food packets contain increasingly empty spaces, and reduced levels of nutritious food; and everywhere we see cheaper processes coming into use. High profit margins and low costs matter above all.

One of the major products of the food industry is fat. It was one of the most important by-products of the beef trade. Carcases were treated to collect the fat. Large amounts could be trimmed off, and the rest was extracted with heat and solvents. Hydrocarbon liquids (rather like dry-cleaning fluid) were used to remove all traces of fat from the remains of a carcase. The solvent was then removed with heat. This fat commanded a good price on world markets. During the 1970s the price of fat fell steadily. The application of heat to sterilize animal wastes is expensive. The cost of using solvents was high, and some solvents are now known to be capable of causing cancer. The meat and bone-meal processing industry sought to have the regulations relaxed so that they could gradually install newer plant which eliminated these processing stages. The quest for deregulation required action at the highest level of government.

There are many manufacturers who would like to claim the sympathy of a senior spokesman for their cause, and in this instance the processors had a direct line of potential sympathy from the Prime Minister herself. Margaret Thatcher was an active proponent of what she saw as an open market economy. Her greatest legacy was a move away from altruism towards the commercialism we still associate with those so-called market forces. In reality this high-sounding principle often amounts to little more than greed.

In Britain during 1980 there was pressure for the deregulation of the animal feed industry. A disastrous explosion at the massive chemical works at Flixborough several years before added weight to those who asked for the use of solvents to be curtailed. By 1982 the costly processing of animal feeds was short-circuited. The use of solvents was dropped, and heat treatment was much reduced. Infective agents like scrapie – which may have been inactivated by the process – would be more likely to survive a gentler form of processing. Infective agents could lie in wait in the animal meal, ready to trigger the most costly episode in the history of agriculture.

It has to be said that nobody could have known this at the time. The short cuts in the processing of animal foodstuffs was meant to save money, not make animals ill. However, though the reduction in the extent of processing saved a substantial percentage in production costs, these savings were not passed on to the consumer. Farmers were told nothing of how the feed was prepared. All they knew was the percentage of protein contained in each batch, with no indication of where it came from. They ended paying roughly as much for the feed, whilst the producers put the added profit straight into their coffers. It is a typical story of our time.

First Cases

Within a couple of years the symptoms of something similar to sheep scrapie had begun to appear in British cattle. One early case was said to be a cow in Hampshire who died mysteriously and was buried in a field. The official response to the new disease was intriguing. The first I heard of it was in 1987. I mentioned that it sounded very like what I knew of scrapie, and the response was, 'We are advised not to compare the two. The use of the term "scrapie" is not encouraged when we are discussing BSE.' It was one of those instant denials that make one wonder whether there is something going on. My belief is that the lowered requirement for sterilization of cattle feed had some great minds almost waiting for trouble. The specialists (who knew of scrapie very well, of course) seemed anxious to divert attention from the possibility of an association. It was the first intimation that there might be collusion to keep the facts under wraps.

In April 1987 a committee had been set up under the chairmanship of Sir Richard Southwood, a distinguished professor at Oxford University. Their conclusions were published by the Department of Health under the title *Report of the Working Party on BSE* in 1989 (Chapter 8). During the previous year they had already issued interim conclusions, recommending that BSE-infected cattle should be destroyed, and their milk discarded.

The *Veterinary Record* published the first report on the incidence of BSE on 31 October 1987. Four cattle herds were said to be infected, as far apart as Kent and Cornwall. One herd had ten cases, the others had one each. The age of the affected cattle was between three and six years. Later surveys tried to collate evidence from even earlier. These retrospective surveys have not proved to be reliable. For instance, the Ministry of Agriculture, Fisheries and Food (MAFF) originally concluded that there were seven cases in 1986. By 1990 they said that the 1986 number of cases had actually been over sixty.

Matters seemed to come to a head when Dr Tom Holt and a dietician, J. Phillips, published a note in the *British Medical Journal* on 4 June 1988. They made a brave suggestion that BSE might pose a risk to humans. My reaction was the same as yours would be: this is a new disease, and we must eradicate it before it takes hold. There are parallels with conditions like blue ear disease of pigs, and foot-and-mouth disease of cattle; in these cases draconian measures are taken to eliminate the infection at its source. Do not believe that this was not the general scientific view: many of the scientists working on the problem felt this was the correct answer, too.

Kill the Beast

A policy of eliminating infected cattle through slaughter was introduced in the summer of 1988, and the suspect meat and bone-meal was banned as well. There was a serious error in the Government's reasoning. Although

BSE was made a notifiable disease in November 1988, farmers were given no financial incentive to report it. If they brought in a cow with BSE they lost money. They still do. As a result, every time a case was found, the canny farmer quickly sent her to market in order to claim full market price. To this day, cows infected with BSE are being sold to farms all over Britain. Many thousands have been sold abroad in recent years.

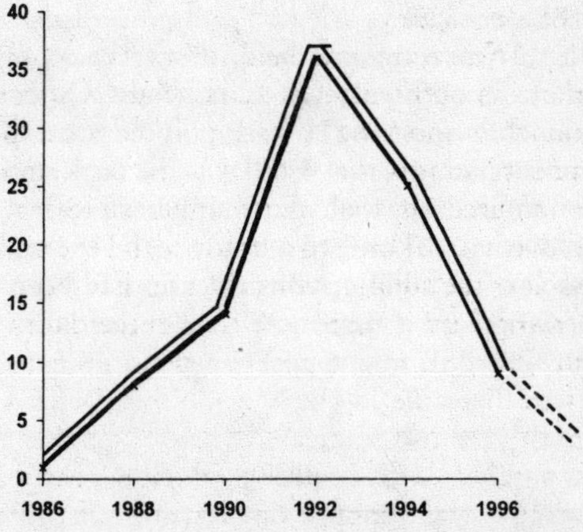

Fig 2: The Rise and Fall of BSE in Britain

The outbreak of new cases of spongy-brain disease, a new strain of kuru, came near the end of the epidemic of BSE in British cattle. Original forecasts said the peak would be reached by 1990, but numbers kept climbing until 1992.

Getting to grips with the truth was not easy. In 1990, as Chairman of the History Sector at the Institute of Biology in London, I chaired the first-ever meeting on the history of BSE. I proposed then that farmers should be offered a bounty for every case they could find. If they were able to make money, rather than lose it, the cattle would be mopped up rapidly. BSE had been made a notifiable disease in June 1988; within two months the slaughter of a diseased animal was compulsory, yet a price of only 50 per cent of the healthy carcase value was paid to the unfortunate farmer who brought her in. Not until 1990 was that raised to 100 per cent. There is still a bonus paid to cows that are BSE-free. My bounty proposal would offer the extra to farmers whose cattle proved BSE-*positive*.

When this meeting was held, it was being officially stated that the outbreak was at its height. On breakfast television that morning I had pointed out that the Government had said that 1990 was the peak; from now on they assured us that the number of cases would steadily diminish. This proved not to be the case. The previous year the total number of cases had been 5,470; the following year it rose more than threefold to nearly 18,000.

Age	1989	1991
2	28	46
3	586	3000
4	2138	7143
5	1874	4680
6	667	2021
7	125	775
8	37	202
9+	15	126
Total	5,470	17,993

Table 1: Age of onset of BSE in Cattle around 1990

There never was a bounty to encourage all animals to be brought in for elimination from the food supply, and now the numbers are too great for the idea to be attractive to government. BSE isn't contagious, as far as we can tell, and we now know the use of such incentives to bring in infected animals would not necessarily have prevented new cases elsewhere. They would be contracting the condition from their feed, not from other cows.

But cattle brought to the attention of the veterinary or public health authorities are not so likely to enter the human food supply, whereas slightly sick cows that are sent for conventional slaughter will soon end up in pies, pasties, sausages or sold as steak. What we need to do is distinguish between the infected cattle and those free of disease. The aim must be to keep the infected cattle out of the human food supply.

Brussels has kept a vigilant eye on BSE. On 18 July 1994 the European Union agriculture ministers agreed to ban the export of carcases from Britain unless they came from a herd which could document that no cases of BSE had been reported in the previous six years. The recent actions are the latest in a long line of continuing regulations. In some ways the EU ministers have been more realistic in their responses than the British government's continual ducking and weaving.

Dairy farms that have had BSE	59.2 percent
Beef herds that have had BSE	15.2 per cent
Adult herds have had BSE	35.5 per cent
Average weekly suspect cases* Spring 1996	279
Average weekly suspect cases* Spring 1995	395
159,122 confirmed cases in total on 33,319 farms	

**For both totals, roughly 15 per cent will prove negative*

Table 2: Incidence of BSE in Britain – April 1996

There have been over 170,000 cases of BSE in British cattle, and details of them all are stored on computer at the Central Veterinary Laboratory in Surrey.

Yet, while the scientific findings have been methodically acquired, the official response has been hasty and ill-considered. The solution offered is that all cattle over a specified age should be eliminated from the food supply. This is an example of the same false reasoning which put us into the position in which we find ourselves. It is reaction by cover-up. The argument behind it is this:

- Young cattle do not manifest the signs and symptoms of BSE
- These animals could be legitimately sold as 'BSE-free'
- The disease usually appears after the age of thirty months
- In cattle, the second teeth normally appear just before this time
- If cattle are slaughtered before the second incisors erupt we can claim that BSE has disappeared

The motivation is: 'cover up and carry on as normal'. This is foolish and short-sighted. It is a commercial decision typical of those with short-term expediency in mind. It may *mask* the existence of BSE, but does nothing to eliminate it. The symptoms may be largely eliminated by this ruse, but the disease itself is not. This debate rumbled on throughout the spring of 1996, with the British authorities railing against the Brussels bureaucrats who would not give a clean bill of health to meat produced under such a scheme.

Brussels was right. This is a cover-up. It is typical of the way decisions are often taken in the 1990s, for it is unscientific and deceitful. It is dishonest because it serves only to hide the extent of the problem, and is unscientific for several reasons.

The age at which these second teeth come through is normally two years three months (twenty-seven months) but the signs in the gums that teeth are due vary from one animal to another, and the farming world is not convinced that the eruption of the teeth is always a reliable indicator of age. The regulations state that the diagnostic feature is 'any sign' of the teeth coming through. Some people interpret that to mean the whiteness of the teeth, others point out that a 'sign' is reddening of the gums. In any event, no-one doubts that a cow free of BSE symptoms at thirty months may be incubating the disease (and infectious) all the while.

Meanwhile, animals which have been reared on grass and are in excellent health will all be excluded from the food supply. There are thousands of them, all just past the thirty-month age barrier. Devoted farmers who have raised them safely could lose hundreds of pounds for every animal they have nurtured, which could be taken away to be shot and burnt.

Taking Urgent Action

Slaughtering herds that are free from BSE, just for the sake of appearances, is a travesty of policy-making and should never have been considered. The only intelligent answer is a targeted policy which eliminates every diseased animal. It is as simple as that. Beef herds are far less likely to contract BSE. There can be arguments about the slaughter of individual animals known to be infected, or the culling of entire herds. One view is that herds where there are six or more cases should be eliminated. This is a matter where specialist advice is vital, and where open debate is necessary.

It is easy to imagine your response – let's just get rid of the lot! It must be said that, if the Government had heeded sensible advice rather than listening to the demands of short-term expediency, then none of this would have been necessary. But that's in the past. We do need to plan ahead, and consider what to do next. Slaughtering the entire British cattle population would be a costly process:

- Farmers were able to claim up to £865 per BSE cow slaughtered
- The present cattle population of Britain totals 12 million
- The total that the Treasury would pay to farmers is £10,380 million – over ten billion pounds
- Disposal of each carcase costs £125
- This additional cost, nationwide, would be £1,500m – one and a half billion pounds
- The British Meat and Livestock Commission estimates there are 400,000 people working in the beef and dairy business
- Every million out of work costs £2,750m (the best part of three billion pounds)
- The total cost of social security would total £1.1m

The losses to industries which handle the beef downstream from the farmers might be mediated, for they could switch to non-British beef to maintain supplies. The total initial cost of these measures (the most expensive scenario imaginable) would be about £14 billion, and the run-on costs might be less than £1 billion a year thereafter. There is the added problem of the additional incinerators we would need, and of course the loss of British milk through the elimination of the national herd which produces it.

In matters of public health, we must always work out the cost of the worst possible situation. We should try to resist panic measures, of course, but start to think things through. For example, farming lobbyists have said that farmers ought to be paid compensation for their lost stock, and then provided with new cattle to take their place. Hold hard, there; that would mean they would be receiving compensation twice over! Britain has been assured of compensation from the European Union to

1985	April	Colin Whitaker reports unrecognized disease
1986	November	First case formally identified
1987	December	British scientists admit they are baffled
1988	April	Sir Richard Southwood sets up Committee
1988	June	BSE a notifiable disease
—	July	Ban on ruminant feed for ruminants
—	August	Compulsory slaughter with 50% compensation
—	December	BSE milk banned (except for cow's own calf)
—	—	Scrapie-contaminated offal blamed
—	—	BSE and CJD – first link postulated
1989	February	Export of cattle born before July '88 banned
1989	November	Specified offal* ban from cattle over 6 months
1990	January	American military bases ban British beef
—	February	100 per cent compensation offered
—	March	First cases in British zoo animals
—	April	Russia bans imports of British beef
—	May	Sir Donald Acheson, Chief Medical Officer of Health, says: 'Beef is absolutely safe to eat.'
—	June	23 non-EU countries ban British beef imports
1994	November	Offal ban includes thymus and gut from calves
1995	August	Stephen Churchill (19) and Maurice Callaghan (30) die from new form of disease
1996	March	Ban on meat and bone-meal for all farm animals

** Includes brain, spinal cord, spleen and thymus, tonsils and intestines*

Table 3: Landmark Dates in BSE

help cover the cost, and it is a traditional ploy for farmers to try to obtain the most money they can from the faceless bureaucrats in Brussels, but we must try to make our plans for the future more reliable than our schemes of the past.

Examining a Slaughter Policy

The wholesale slaughter of all cattle above a certain age at this stage is ill-considered and pointless. The epidemic of BSE in cattle is now on the wane. We were recording over 1,000 new cases a week when the outbreak was at its highest, and now the figure is 250 per week. Targeted slaughter eliminates the BSE-infected cattle, whereas a wholesale mass killing would be a foolish tragedy.

Farmers have spent years (generations, sometimes) building up their herds. Many of these animals have never been near meat and bone-meal. The loss of their treasured cattle would be a terrible blow, and it is an unnecessary measure to impose. If wholesale slaughter were to be introduced, irrespective of the health of the herd, then the cattle would not be the only ones to die.

3

VOICES FROM THE PAST

Scrapie is a strange name. It has simple origins, for it refers to the way infected sheep scrape themselves against walls and posts as they try to relieve the itching they must feel. Scrapie is an old affliction, and has been well-known in sheep for centuries. The first cases in the English-speaking world probably occurred in Merino sheep imported from Spain in the fifteenth century. Since then it has been given a variety of names – 'animal rickets', for example. It has even been dubbed 'distemper', which is a disease of domestic animals and has no relationship to scrapie. By 1759 it was known as the 'trotting disease' to German investigators. In 1811 the French recognized it as the 'malady of madness and convulsions', and more recently have called it *la tremblante*. There is a condition grandly known as Paraplexia Enzootica Ovium, which is also really scrapie.

1732 is the date when the disease was clinically recognized in Britain; but it was the beautifully written article by Leopold in Germany in 1759 which gave the first classical description:

> 'Some sheep also suffer from scrapie, which can be identified by the fact that the animals lie down, bite at their feet and legs, rub their back against posts, fail to thrive, stop feeding, and finally become lame . . . This illness is incurable. The best solution, therefore, is for the shepherd to dispose of a suffering sheep quickly, slaughtering it away from the manorial lands. A shepherd must isolate such an animal away from the healthy stock immediately, for it is infectious and can cause serious harm in the flock.'

Scrapie in Britain during the late eighteenth century was described in a book in which Dr Parry lists the precautions shepherds used to take. His advice matches our current understanding of scrapie very well. The disease was the first spongiform encephalopathy to be recognized. It is interesting that the finest description came from Germany, for that is a country which now claims to have no cases of scrapie at all. In 1799 the Bath and West of England Society journal published an account of the diagnosis of scrapie in sheep. Shepherds were even advised to prevent the ewe from devouring the placenta after birth, a practice since followed by farmers raising cattle.

In 1789 the Highland Society published a detailed account of sheep which showed scrapie was still absent from that region; it was not in Scotland until 1850. By the middle of the nineteenth century, scrapie was found as far east as the River Danube, as far south as Spain, as far west as the Atlantic coast. Sometimes there were epidemics. Between 1750 and 1820 there were extensive outbreaks in Britain, and from 1780 there was an epidemic in Germany which lasted twenty years.

In most of Britain, the incidence of scrapie died down late in the nineteenth century but it has slowly increased again during the 1900s. It has since been reported right across Europe, for example in Holland, Italy, Switzerland and Spain. It is present in Japan. In several other countries it has begun to spread after being imported in infected animals: Iceland, Norway and Cyprus, for example. The condition is absent from Australasia, and has never occurred in other countries including Argentina and Uruguay.

What Causes Scrapie?

There were many theories as to the cause. The changing hypotheses have mirrored the fashionable scientific preoccupations of the time, as theories often do. Currently we are in an era which is concerned about pollution and the environment, so it is inevitable that some theories about the origin of BSE should concern pesticides and the agricultural use of chemicals. In the mid nineteenth century the focus of cultural concern was moral welfare and sexual control. Thus in 1848 it was suggested that scrapie was a mental degeneration caused by sexual excess in libidinous animals. As electricity came to the knowledge of the general public, and electrical therapy was a current fashion more than a hundred years ago, it was soon being claimed that scrapie resulted from a high-voltage discharge of lightning.

As the nineteenth century went by, high-resolution microscopes were becoming popular. With these instruments available, science entered the era of 'brass and glass'. Many specialists began to look at tissue preparations from animals who had died of diseases of the brain. In 1899 French scientists discovered the spongy degeneration of the nervous tissues so characteristic of these diseases. In fact, French and German scientists led the way in research into scrapie well into the twentieth century.

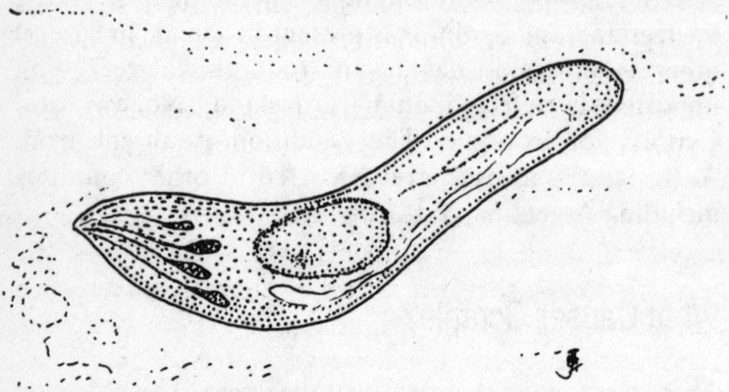

Fig 3: Sarcocystis
This tiny organism, almost big enough to be seen with the naked eye, is sometimes found in sheep. Early research workers found it in sections of tissue from victims of scrapie, and believed it could cause the disease. However, we now know that Sarcocystis *also occurs in sheep free of scrapie, and is absent from many of the confirmed cases. It cannot be the cause.*

Finding the microscopical evidence of the disease is one thing; determining the cause is another matter altogether. One of the early theories was that the disease was caused by a germ. One candidate for the 'germ of scrapie' was *Sarcocystis,* a microscopic parasite of animals. This has been found to cause disease in cattle and pigs (only rarely in humans) but it usually has little effect on the host. The only time symptoms appear is if the tiny germs get into a major organ, like the pancreas or the brain. A belief that *Sarcocystis* caused scrapie is not as far-fetched as some of the earlier theories. If the germ gets to the brain, tiny cysts form and they are similar to the vacuoles of spongy-brain disease. Not only that, but there are no signs of inflammation around the damaged areas. There is no inflammation in scrapie or BSE, either. As a rule you expect to find inflammation wherever there is an invading germ, because this is the body's way of rejecting the parasite. The fact that inflammation was not found in *Sarcocystis* infections gives it something else in common with scrapie.

In time this theory had to be abandoned. Scrapie was observed to occur in animals where there was no *Sarcocystis*, and the little microbe was detected in other animals that were free of scrapie. It is still possible that germs like *Sarcocystis* could carry an infective agent into the body of a new host, and even into the brain, but there is no reason to believe that this germ actually causes scrapie.

During 1918 the Principal of the Royal Veterinary College carried out a series of experiments to see how the disease might be transmitted from one host to another. He also spent much time examining the internal organs of animals which had died of scrapie. None of his techniques worked reliably, but he did make one important observation: namely, that the incubation period of the disease seemed to be very long. He believed that this was a serious problem which needed to be addressed. Before long, scientists were discussing the safety question – was meat from sheep infected with scrapie a risk to people who ate it?

An Imaginary Breakthrough

Then in 1926 came a dramatic breakthrough, or so it seemed at the time. An eminent researcher, Sir Stuart Stockman, reported in volume 39 of the *Journal of Comparative Pathology* that he had observed the recovery to full health of several sheep who had suffered severely from scrapie. He then spoilt it rather by adding that his extensive studies of brain specimens from these animals showed that they did not have any signs of the spongy appearance everyone else had observed. It later turned out that he was mistaken; his 'recovered' sheep had never suffered from scrapie at all.

By this stage there was a growing body of knowledge on scrapie. It was becoming clear that this was an insidious disease, and it would not follow the rules which applied elsewhere in microbiology. The next problem was to find out how it spread. The *Sarcocystis* theory had been launched at a time when bacteria and other microscopic germs were being found to cause a range of infections. By the time of the Second World War, the focus was on the newly-recognized virus diseases. It was known that you couldn't study them with a conventional microscope, but you could still study their effects.

The Vaccine which brought Death

The first time that scrapie had been shown to be transmissible was in the 1930s, when a new vaccine was introduced. It was designed to prevent outbreaks of louping-ill in sheep, an inflammation of the brain spread by ticks. The vaccine had been sterilized with formalin. This is a powerful disinfectant, but still not strong enough to inactivate the agents of spongy-brain diseases like scrapie. As a result, doses of scrapie were injected with the vaccination and hundreds of sheep went down with the disease.

Two diligent French microbiologists named Cuillé and Chelle took this further, and in 1936 they found that they could transfer specimens from the spinal cord of infected animals, to produce scrapie in sheep. This was painstaking work, for they found that the incubation period of the disease was very different from that of any known virus infection. Virus diseases take hold in a few days, as a rule, whilst the scrapie infection took between one and two years to appear. This was a vital advance. In 1942 the two Frenchmen made another breakthrough. This time they proved that scrapie was not confined to sheep, and they detected it in a goat.

A Scientist Laughed to Scorn

One percipient research worker during the 1940s lost his reputation because of his enthusiasm. He was Dr D. R. Wilson, who was fascinated by the disease. He showed that serum, even after being filtered free of the tiniest solid particles, could still transmit the disease – so it was clearly not caused by a bacterium. He went on to show that the infective agent was not destroyed by formalin, and that it was amazingly resistant to heat – so it did not seem to be a virus, either. He noted these observations, and then went on to transmit the scrapie agent through nine successive sheep, which proved that the agent could keep its infectivity, and which further substantiated its unique properties.

As the evidence began to accrue, it became clear that this was no ordinary illness. It was confirmed that the infective agent, whatever it was, could resist high temperatures. Even the autoclave (a laboratory version of the domestic pressure-cooker) did not inactivate it, though cooking at those temperatures kills even the most resistant bacterial spores and inactivates all known viruses. Because normal disinfectants had little effect, it was difficult to sterilize equipment when working with scrapie.

These were important discoveries, and they implied that science was faced with a wholly new form of infection. Wilson's research was before its time, and he was belittled because of it. Nobody was willing to believe the evidence he had published. It cost him his reputation, and the fact that he turned out to have been right came too late to save his honour.

By this time, there was a growing body of evidence to support these revolutionary views. Clearly, there was something strange about the agent that causes scrapie. It had none of the properties of any conventional germ, and produced a disease which was untreatable and always killed its victims. It also took a long time to appear. What could this strange agent be?

Birth of a Slow Virus

The next reasonable explanation arose in Iceland. A veterinary researcher, Björn Sigurdsson, came up with the new idea of 'slow viruses'. He brought together several diseases found in Icelandic sheep, including *maedi* (a lung disease), *visna* (a nervous complaint), *jaagziegte* (infectious lung cancer caused by a virus) and *rida* (scrapie). He saw they had several key factors in common:

- Infections were usually confined to a single organ, not spread through the body
- Very long incubation period (years, in many cases)
- A slowly degenerative course
- Invariably fatal outcome

This 'slow virus' idea attracted much interest. There were many chronic, long-term diseases which fitted into the category, including one in humans very like BSE in cattle. This is the exceedingly rare Gerstmann-Sträußler-Scheinker syndrome, known as GSS for short. Sadly, the idea did not stand up to scrutiny. These diseases had no clinical features in common, their causes seemed to be a mixed bunch, and the few which were thought to be caused by viruses were associated with viruses of very different types. The factors they had in common turned out to be no more than coincidence.

Research on scrapie was proceeding modestly, until an audacious research programme in 1957. It was the 'Twenty-Four Breed Experiment', and showed that scrapie existed in several different forms. It also established that the genetic susceptibility to scrapie varied with the breed. A huge sample of 1,027 sheep were injected with scrapie agent on a single day. As the title of the experiment showed, they were selected from twenty-four different breeds of all shapes and sizes. There were between thirty and fifty-seven sheep in each breed, and they were kept for two years and carefully monitored. The results gave us the first large database on susceptibility to scrapie.

A completely new idea arose during the 1950s. This proposed that scrapie was not a disease of the nervous system at all, but was essentially a disease of muscle. Studies with the microscope seemed to confirm the suspicion. But a detailed study in 1958 showed that, even though you could see muscles degenerate as the scrapie progressed, the disease was centred on the nervous system. It was clear that it was highly infectious, for Dr Iain Pattison showed that samples of placenta from Swaledale ewes could pass the disease to other sheep and goats. The sheep and goats were shown to become infected through eating placental tissues, as they sometimes did in the wild. This gave one major reason why scrapie was so widespread in nature.

These observations were taking a long time to make, and it was clear that far more would be learned if only there was a simple way to carry out observations. In 1961 a crucial step was taken when a scientist, Dr Dickinson, showed that scrapie could be transferred to mice. It then turned out to infect hamsters as well. Scrapie does not naturally occur in either of these species. It is now known that there are over twenty 'strains' of scrapie. Some produce a version of the disease in which animals become drowsy and inactive (in at least one form the animal victims simply drop dead without prior warning), whilst others cause an illness where the animals can't stop scratching. Some develop quickly, others are slow. Many of the experimental results now available, some of which may help us to understand the human varieties of these diseases, are most surprising.

For example, what do you suppose happens if an animal receives an inoculation of a 'fast' and a 'slow' strain of scrapie in a mixed dose? The disease with the shortest incubation time is always the one which appears. It is as though the two agents are competing, and the one which develops more quickly seizes an advantage. Very well, so what happens if an animal has a dose of a 'slow' strain first, and a dose of a 'fast' strain later? In this case the disease develops slowly. Clearly, even if the 'fast' strains have some advantages, they are kept in the background once the 'slow' version has taken hold. We have no real explanations for these phenomena.

Scrapie is a terrible disease. Mercifully, sheep are usually slaughtered before the symptoms appear. The agent is known to mutate – an extraordinary fact, bearing in mind that it isn't an organism, or even a virus. It is known to pass from ewes to their lambs by infection through the placenta, and from one adult animal to another through feeding on infected remains. How does the agent get to the brain? It seems to pass from the gut to the spleen through the blood supply. The spleen has a nervous connection to the spinal cord, and it may be that the agent passes to the brain through this splanchnic nerve. In support of this theory is the observation that, if you remove the spleen from a newly infected animal, the disease takes much longer to appear in the central nervous system.

A test for scrapie has been hard to envisage. Once the agent has entered the body it disappears for a time. When it does reappear it is typically in the spleen, and by the time it can be traced to the brain the incubation period is already halfway gone. We now believe that diseases like scrapie are related to strange proteins called prions which can produce diseased cells (Chapter 14). They have begun to emerge in many different species, and may now be set to face us with a new and fascinating problem as we welcome a new millennium. As human victims of new spongy-brain diseases are recorded, many of the insights we need have been gained from the inquisitive workers of the past. Their studies of sheep, mice and hamsters are the basis of our current understanding. Without those pioneers of the past we would be faced with a future of intimidating mystery.

4

WHOSE BRAIN GETS SPONGY?

Not every type of animal has been shown to develop this type of illness. Some seem immune. The spongy-brain diseases have almost always been found solely in mammals, and then only in some groups of mammals. It may be that the conditions are found in other types of animal. A strange form of spongiform encephalopathy has recently turned up in the bird kingdom too. The birds are a bridge between mammals and the vast world of reptiles. If the findings in birds are confirmed, then the spongy-brain diseases may be more widespread than we thought.

When scrapie was first transmitted to rodents it caused much surprise. Scrapie was a disease of sheep. Yes, it had been found in goats too, but they are closely related. These are all animals which chew the cud and have cleft feet. We call them ruminants. Rats, mice and hamsters are rodents, and they are a different class. This term comes from the Latin for 'gnaw', and that's what they spend much of their lives doing. Small animals like this have often been used to study human disease and to help search for a cure. The fact that scrapie could be transmitted to rodents has taught us many lessons.

- First, it provides a useful laboratory model in which we can study the disease.
- Second, it shows that this strange disease can be passed into groups of animals that have never known it before.
- Thirdly, it provides the only viable test we have for the infectivity of the agent of scrapie.

These simple statements provide good news, and bad. The good news is that an animal model which can be studied might tell us much about the progress of the illness and its way of attacking the nervous system. We need that to understand what is going on, and to work towards medical answers to these potential problems.

The second conclusion, however, has a worrying implication. It was believed that scrapie was somehow confined to sheep and their closest allies. If human intervention could pass the disease to different animal groups where it had been completely unknown, this also shows that spongy-brain disease could pose a greater danger than we thought. Much has been made of the belief that the BSE agent jumped the 'species barrier' into people. It should have surprised no-one. People themselves had already made it jump the species barrier into mice.

Had People caught Scrapie?

It was never felt that there was much risk to people from scrapie. It has been around for centuries. As far as we knew, nobody had ever caught it. Lamb is known as a particularly innocuous meat – it has been said that it's the one form of meat to which people are never allergic – and it is a staple food for many semi-arid countries. In the

Arab lands it is normal for a family to take a pet lamb to the desert or the shore for a picnic. The children run in the waves or the sand, the parents chat around a barbecue, the *shisha* is lit and handed around as the bubbles of smoke pass through rose-water in a great glass globe, the sheep is petted and fed some scraps of local vegetation. When it is time for the meal the sheep is untethered and brought across and then, with a knife as well-honed as a scalpel, its throat is cut and within minutes it is grilling on the charcoal embers and browning in the heat. You won't find fresher cooked meat anywhere.

Perhaps your eye was caught by comments on scrapie in a previous paragraph: 'nobody had ever caught it', I wrote. Could that be true? Perhaps the human spongy-brain condition now called Creutzfeldt-Jakob disease (CJD) is the human equivalent of scrapie. Sufferers may not share all the symptoms clearly suffered by sheep, but the tiny cavities in the brain are much the same, and the fatal outcome is closely similar.

This is not a new idea. When CJD and the other forms of spongy-brain disease were first recognized it was natural to speculate that people might be catching scrapie from sheep. For all the medical similarities, there was one strong argument against the idea. The finding was that only one person in a million develops a spongy-brain disease in a typical community. There were some areas where the number was higher (there was a cluster in Libya, for example, which proved to have a genetic cause).

Creutzfeldt-Jakob disease

Apart from local concentrations, the ratio of CJD cases was one in a million wherever one looked. This applied to countries where scrapie was widespread, and it was also true in countries where there was no scrapie at all. The reasoning is clear. If scrapie was being passed to people, you'd expect that the number of cases of human spongy-brain disease would rise in areas where scrapie was abundant, and would fall to zero where there was no chance of exposure. It was this reasoning that led many policy-makers to feel confident that, if scrapie wasn't passed to humans, then BSE would not bridge the gap either.

They should have remembered that it could be passed to rodents. Before long, spongy-brain disease was next reported in cats; some domestic, others big cats in zoos. It is now believed that this came from feed carrying a scrapie-like infection. It has even been observed in ostriches, though nobody has shown that this form is infectious. None the less, these are potentially disturbing findings. A disease agent that is confined to ruminants is one thing, but an agent that can spread to rodents, to carnivores, and even to birds as well, paints a much more threatening picture.

Scrapie

This disease remains the baseline from which all other studies have stemmed. Scrapie is widespread around the world. Some areas are naturally unaffected (including some South American states) while others are kept free by government decree (including Australia and New Zealand). Other areas have official controls but do next to nothing about it (including the European Union).

Both sexes of sheep are affected, and the disease is found in most breeds. The average age at which the disease reaches its peak is three and a half years. At first the symptoms are few and the start of the disease is hard to observe. Experienced shepherds can spot it earlier than scientific observers. One of the first signs is that the fleece feels different to the touch, being harsher and less soft than normal. It is a small change, but characteristic of the disease, and a wise shepherd can detect it at once.

The infected sheep tend to take less exercise as the disease establishes its hold. They walk unsteadily, and drink small amounts of water at frequent intervals. They pass urine in small amounts, and more frequently than normal. The skin becomes irritated, so they scratch against fences and walls.

This behaviour is not always found in every version of scrapie. The Icelandic strain of scrapie known locally as *rida* traditionally caused relatively little skin irritation, for scraping and scratching by the sick sheep were rarely seen in Iceland. But the infection is changing; skin irritation was almost never seen in Icelandic sheep with scrapie, but in recent years this symptom has started to appear. It is now frequently seen. Spongy-brain disease is changing with time.

As the disease progresses the sheep behave differently. They seem more nervous, anxious almost, and may become uncharacteristically aggressive. Often they leave the flock and wander off on their own. They show extra sensitivity to touch or sound. It is interesting to see how the characteristic symptoms in each area are reflected in the regional name for the disease. Sheep with scrapie in France often develop a twitch or tremor in the muscles, which explains the French name for the disease, *la tremblante*. In Germany a frequent sign is abnormal movement by trotting or hopping rather like a rabbit, with both hind legs together. Not surprisingly, the German name for the disease is *Der Traberkrankheit*, literally 'the trotting illness'.

In different breeds of sheep, and at different times, scrapie has shown itself to be a varied range of similar diseases. Since we have recognized the existence of mad cow disease, there has been no noteworthy change in scrapie seen in sheep or goats. The age of onset and the clinical signs remain unaltered. Scrapie is not necessarily the agent which caused BSE by spreading to cattle.

There are many mysteries still in store, however; one strange version of scrapie found in Shetland results in sheep dropping dead, with few if any signs beforehand. No matter what it takes, the pattern of symptoms paints a distressing picture and scrapie causes much suffering to sheep. Research work is needed to find a permanent answer to this burden of suffering for our animal stocks. It should always be remembered that scientific research finds cures for animal diseases, as well as for those that afflict people.

There are many forms of spongy-brain disease now recognized in the animal world. Not all of them are infectious, but they are more varied and widespread than has been generally reported. Let us go through them and set out the state of scientific knowledge in each case.

Wasting Disease of Deer

Naturalists in North America have long been aware of a similar disease of the deer family. It is known as chronic wasting disease (CWD) and it has been seen in deer and elk. The first outbreak was recorded in 1980 at a wildlife centre in Colorado. Later it was seen in Wyoming, in colonies of deer born and raised in captivity. If we consider the signs and symptoms you can see how it seems strangely similar to scrapie, though it differs in detail.

Deer with CWD go to drink water much more frequently than normal. About 15 per cent of deer with CWD die of pneumonia caused by a build-up of water in the gullet and rumen, which literally overflows into the lungs. These sick deer pass urine at abnormally frequent intervals, much as you might expect. They lose weight, and behave abnormally towards keepers or other animals in a herd. Elk are less often seen to have abnormal drinking behaviour, but they frequently develop skin irritation (which is much less common in the deer with the disease). This condition has never been observed outside North America. Nobody knows where this disease originated, but it may be an ancient disease of the deer family, just as scrapie has a long history in sheep.

Sick Mink

In mink we have a condition which has almost certainly originated from an agent causing spongy-brain disease in other animals. It is known as transmissible mink encephalopathy, TME (which means, in English, infectious mink brain disease). As the mink become ill, they change their normal behaviour. This is an insidious process, hard to recognize as they are aggressive at the best of times. The mink become over-excitable and react even to slight noises they'd normally ignore. Then they start to become less clean in their habits. Normally fastidious when they pass their droppings, they become careless and dirty. Keepers notice that they are reluctant to climb up the cage to collect food from the top; mink are naturally active creatures and normally like to do that.

As the disease progresses they start to hunch up, drawing the tail over the back like a squirrel's. They creep about, often biting at the tail apparently to relieve itching. Sometimes they mutilate themselves by biting severely. They hold onto objects – for instance, they will grip a stick so strongly they can be lifted up from the floor. They may linger on for a month, but in many outbreaks they die within a week. Where did TME originate? This is a disease which is only found in farmed mink, and has never been reported in any wild animals. Scrapie is an obvious likely cause, for farmed mink have long been fed meal containing waste sheep-meat.

However, this easy answer cannot be the complete answer. Many American mink farms have never fed any meal containing sheep products. Mink are carnivorous animals, and need meat in the diet, but many farms exclusively feed waste from the slaughter of cattle and have never had access to meal contaminated with scrapie. One well-studied outbreak occurred in a farm where old 'downer cows' were the source of food for the mink. None of the cows had ever shown signs of BSE, but they may have passed the agent to the mink. If true, what could this mean? Only one thing: that the cattle were suffering from a low-grade form of spongy-brain disease which didn't actually produce any clinical signs, but which could run riot in its new host.

Or perhaps not . . . since this form of feed has been used in other mink farms where there have never been any outbreaks of the disease. Evidence could come from experiments to transmit BSE to mink and, yes, this has been done. These experimentally infected animals do develop disease, but its effects are different from those in classical TME. The whole affair is confusing, and the evidence is contradictory. Though a fuller understanding is clearly within reach, we are not there yet.

Do Zoo Animals develop BSE?

The range of infected animals is far greater than it was. To the sheep and goats we can now add such majestic animals as the Arabian oryx and the greater kudu. The gemsbok and the eland have also been found with it.

Among the great cats are the cheetah and the puma, together with a recent case in an ocelot. All these cases arose in British zoos. The few that are now outside British shores were infected in Britain and then exported.

The first findings were published in 1995 by a committee headed by Dr David Tyrrell, who pioneered virus research at the Common Cold Research centre in Wiltshire for many years. James Kirkwood, of London Zoo, has kept a count of the outbreaks. As this book goes to press, the total number of cases is twenty-three captive animals belonging to nine separate species. Table 4 (opposite) gives dates of the first of each case.

The first cases to be reported were in animals fed on the same sheep-meal which has been associated with the spread of BSE, and it was believed that the ban imposed on such feed in 1989 would lead to an end to new cases. This did not happen. Some animals born after the ban was imposed have developed the disease. First was a greater kudu, then an eland, and they were followed by a scimitar-horned oryx. The symptoms were generally like those of BSE and scrapie, but the effects varied with the species.

- Kudu are magnificent creatures, amongst the largest of all antelopes, and 1.5 m (5 feet) tall at the shoulder. They are brown or grey, with a broad stripe down the back and fainter stripes down the sides. It is the horns of the male which are the most striking feature about these animals: over a metre (a yard) long, they are thick at the base and spiral to a fine tip. Kudu feed on grass and other leafy vegetation in the wild. The nyala is also a member of this tribe. The zoo animals stricken with spongy-brain disease became listless and started licking their noses. The head was held at an unusual angle, and there was a tremor easily visible as the animals tried to stand still. In these species there was an unexpected variation in the progress of the disease. In two cases the animals collapsed and died within a

Host	Disease	First report	Distribution
Cattle	Bovine spongiform encephalopathy (BSE)	1986	UK, Ireland, France,Switzerland, Oman, Germany Portugal, Canada, Denmark
Nyala	Spongiform encephalopathy (SE)	1987	England
Gemsbok	SE	1988	England
Arabian oryx	SE	1989	England
Greater kudu	SE	1989	England
Eland	SE	1989	England
Cat	Feline SE (FSE)	1990	British Isles
Moufflon	Scrapie	1992	England
Puma	FSE	1992	England
Cheetah	FSE	1992	Australia, Britain, Ireland
Scimitar-horned oryx	SE	1993	England
Ocelot	FSE	1994	England

Table 4: Cases of Infective Spongy-brain diseases reported 1985-1995

day of becoming ill; in the most protracted illness a kudu survived fifty-six days.

- Eland are the biggest of all antelopes, up to 1.8 m (six feet) tall at the shoulder and with spiralling horns at least as long as those of a kudu. The females have horns, though they are far smaller than those of the male. They are gregarious creatures and live for more than twenty years. When spongy-brain disease strikes the animals become jumpy and nervous. They tremble continually, and drool from nose and mouth.
- The scimitar oryx is regarded as an endangered species. It stands a little shorter than the kudu but has gently curved horns that are longer than either of the previous species. When the disease strikes, these creatures also show drooling. The most marked sign is a loss of muscular coordination, and they rapidly lose the ability to walk or even to stand.
- Gemsbok are the best-known species of oryx. The signs they display are similar, though these creatures are particularly liable to collapse, suddenly and without warning.

Many related animals were fed the same feed, and have never shown signs of the disease. It is becoming clear that some species are particularly susceptible to the agent of spongy-brain disease, whilst others seem to resist its attack. In either event, there is surely a strange poignancy about seeing such majestic and elegant creatures struck down by a condition resulting from human mismanagement.

In 1990 a cat went down with feline SE. It caused much public comment at the time, but specialists were not surprised that a cat had contracted spongy-brain disease. Cats had already been shown to be susceptible to the agent of BSE in experiments done in the United States and in Czechoslovakia. The total number of infected cats in Britain reached fifty within just four years. The very name 'feline spongiform encephalopathy' implies that this could be a disease of the *entire* cat family, and so it proved to be. A puma, followed by four cheetahs, contracted FSE. More recently an ocelot and another puma have been added to the list. Although lions and tigers have been fed the same food, they have not been seen to succumb to its effects.

The symptoms are much as you might, by now, expect. The animals cannot groom themselves effectively. They walk with a stooping gait, hold the head at an angle, and dribble constantly. When going to pass urine or faeces they have difficulty in crouching properly, and they tend to lose balance. If a cat leaps on its prey – trying to catch a mouse or bird – it misjudges the distance. The behaviour changes, though not predictably. Some become excessively timid, and try to hide, while others are abnormally aggressive.

What other examples are awaiting discovery? Time alone will reveal the extent of these diseases. However there are some older accounts which we still have to reconcile with current knowledge. Between 1970 and 1977 white tigers were shown to suffer from a degenerative condition of the brain. There is no suggestion that this particular condition was ever infectious.

Bird-Brained Ideas

Ostrich farming could provide one alternative source of meat. Some school caterers already feature ostrich burgers on their menus, and ostrich farming has been touted as a new growth area for investment. As the beef scare reached its climax, the major ostrich farming corporation ceased trading. Investors were apparently willing to invest £20,000 to buy three breeding birds. The birds were apparently kept in Belgium, and the authorities were investigating rumours that the same birds had been 'sold' to more than one owner.

Unknown to these gullible investors, there have already been reports of a spongy-brain disease in ostriches. The cases were reported between 1986 and 1989. Studies of the brain and nervous tissues from ostriches who had succumbed to the disease showed microscopical changes that were much the same as you would expect to find in a case of BSE. I dare say investors might have thought twice about the chance of success had they known of the possibility that the birds may have their own form of spongy-brain disease.

More research is urgently needed, for if spongy-brain diseases can occur in birds too, the problem may be more widespread in nature than anyone had supposed.

5

THE FIRST HUMAN VICTIMS

Papua New Guinea extends for almost half a million square kilometres (180,000 square miles) across the western Pacific. It is twice the size of Britain. Much of the interior is unexplored and, for all its proximity to Australasia, little is still known of the forest tribes. Some of them have yet to be confronted by a European explorer.

The area fascinates explorers because of its beauty and unspoiled forests. During the expeditions into the interior in the 1950s, Western explorers began to learn more about the inhabitants of the Eastern Highlands who were members of the Fore tribe. These Stone Age people were farmers and hunters, and revealed much of the old ways of life. To this day their jungle territories are bursting with unidentified wildlife, and many of the tropical plants may prove to be sources of valuable drugs for the medical needs of a new millennium.

One disease, though, could not be treated by the traditional remedies of the tropical rain forest. The symptoms were a little like malaria. The sufferers would tremble and shiver. They found it difficult to hold objects or to walk. They always got worse. After a few months they could not even stand, and they lay where they were with eyes staring, sometimes grinning insanely yet unable to communicate, until they died. It was a tragic and terrible end.

To the local population it was known as the 'laughing death'. The explorers were told that these poor people were shivering: *kuru* in the local language, so kuru is what the disease is called by Western scientists. It decimated villages. Victims could be seen lolling about, crawling across the floor, or shivering and smiling strangely in their beds.

Science Discovers Kuru

The first scientific accounts of kuru were published by Professor Carleton Gajdusek and Dr V. Zigas in 1957. At first it was believed that the disease was caught from pigs, but later it turned out that cannibalism was rife. It was the cannibalism which was linked to the disease. The victims were in the age range of five to forty years. This was also the range of the incubation period. These tribal people used to celebrate the death of elderly relatives by opening the skull of these newly deceased persons and devouring the brain, or smearing it on their bodies.

More than 2,500 patients died of kuru in the Eastern Highlands of Papua New Guinea between 1957 to 1975. One per cent of the population was lost to the sickness every year. It was a plague as bad as the modern scourge of heart attacks and cancer in the West. By 1960 cannibalism was outlawed, and the incidence of kuru began to subside. One or two cases are still found, but no patient aged under twenty-two years had died since 1973, and no case of kuru has been recorded in anyone born after 1959. It is a matter of calculated guesswork to know whether this is because the incubation period can reach close to fifty years, or whether covert cannibalism still goes on. These time-honoured and deeply ingrained rituals often persist long after official disapproval has been expressed.

During these studies the similarity between kuru and scrapie was noted, and the two diseases were drawn together in a paper for the *Lancet*. A major study of kuru was undertaken by Dr Gajdusek. He lived in the traditional way, among the people, in an extended social group. Regular shipments of brain samples were sent back to the USA. At one stage his activities incurred official disapproval, and he could not obtain entry directly into Papua New Guinea. To carry on his activities he travelled instead to the neighbouring country, Irian Jaya, and walked across the frontier on a little-known track. His first paper appeared in the *New England Journal of Medicine* for 1957. This research brought Dr Gajdusek the Nobel Prize for Medicine in 1976.

Over the following ten years, further experiments with these agents showed that sometimes the infection could easily jump from one species to another. The disease has been induced in primates and also in mink and ferrets. These studies have revealed that there are fourteen strains of kuru, eleven of which have been studied in small rodents (including rats and guinea-pigs). Only three of these strains produced disease in the rodents, so we are faced with a baffling range of agents with differing degrees of danger. The fact that the disease could spread to varied types of animals was an important conclusion. It was also a crucial warning; a warning which governments failed to heed.

The First Spongy-Brain in Humans

Kuru was not the first spongy-brain disease in people to be identified. That dubious distinction goes to Creutzfeldt-Jakob disease which was first described in 1920. Whereas kuru is a disease of the young, CJD does not normally appear prior to the age of forty. There is no known relationship between the classical form of this condition and where people live or what they eat. Like all the other examples, it is invariably fatal and kills by destroying the structure of the brain and central nervous system.

The name of this haunting disease was proposed in 1922. It commemorates two German medical researchers, Dr Creutzfeldt (who recorded the first case in 1920) and Professor Jakob, who made a follow-up study of further patients with the disease. It was Jakob who first recognized that it might be an unusual form of infection of the brain. In 1923 he suggested that it might be possible to transmit the sickness to other animals using brain specimens from patients. This proved to be correct.

Dr W. B. Matthews of Oxford was the first person to attempt an analysis of the frequency with which the disease occurred in the population. He found records of 46 cases of CJD in the period 1964-73 (suggesting 4–5 cases per year), 267 cases between 1970-84 (about 18 cases per year). In the last five years, the recorded rate was put at over 30 cases per year. This does not indicate that the number of actual cases is rising, for the increase is more likely due to greater awareness of the disease. The number of cases for 1995, for example, was rather lower than average. A parallel investigation in France revealed about one case in three million between 1968-1982.

In recent years there have been cases of Creutzfeldt-

Jakob disease which have been passed on through medical treatment. These include:

- Human gonadotrophin
- Human growth hormone
- Corneal grafts in ophthalmic hospitals
- Electrodes experimentally implanted in the brain
- Grafts (injections) of brain cells in degenerative diseases
- Instruments used in surgical operations on the central nervous system

The transmission of CJD by hormones obtained from human organs has led to a ban on the use of hormones extracted from glands (like the pituitary) obtained at post-mortem.

These cases were iatrogenic in origin: they were inadvertently caused by doctors. Such examples have been very rare, for most cases of Creutzfeldt-Jakob disease have no known cause. They may be genetic (some cases are certainly hereditable); they may result from acquisition of an infective agent, but in truth nobody knows why they arise. CJD is different from kuru in several respects. It involves a rapid deterioration, for the disease usually reaches its fatal outcome within three to six months after the symptoms first appear. Dementia is normal in this disease. Patients suffer from loss of memory and intelligence, and they may lose their balance and even become blind. In some patients twitching movements of the limbs become increasingly frequent until they require permanent nursing care. The young are normally spared this wretched illness, for it usually attacks people aged between fifty and seventy-five years.

Gerstmann-Sträußler-Scheinker syndrome

Some people suffer a spongy-brain disorder that comes into a different category. One such rare condition is Gerstmann-Sträußler-Scheinker syndrome, GSS for short. The first case was described by Dr Gerstmann in a medical journal published in Vienna in 1928, and eight years later – with his colleagues Messrs Sträußler and Scheinker – he wrote a lengthy paper on the syndrome for the leading German neurology journal. People in the age range 40-55 years are at risk, and the disease has a longer course than CJD. It can run for over ten years. The microscopical appearance of the brain is also rather different in this disease, which seems to be an inherited condition. It is extremely rare, with one case in every fifty million of the population. Even less well-known is fatal familial insomnia, FFI, which seems to be due to a rare genetic mutation (Chapter 14). Since the middle 1980s, spongy-brain disease of cattle, bovine spongiform encephalopathy or BSE, has been the new addition to this category.

Were People at Risk?

Since 1980 it had been known that these infections could pass across the species barrier, so could it transmit the disease to people? We can learn much by studying the evidence from the areas of the world where the diseases occur. Britain is one area, for BSE has been almost entirely confined to Britain. There are areas where scrapie occurs, and also large areas of the world where scrapie is absent. Most notable are the tracts across Asia and the whole of Australia and New Zealand, where scrapie is not found. It has long been known that the incidence of the human equivalent of

BSE, such as Creutzfeldt-Jakob disease, is as high in the scrapie-free nations as it is in Britain. From this it was assumed that scrapie was not the origin of CJD. If scrapie wasn't, then there was good reason to assume that BSE would not be involved, either.

There was a flaw in the argument, arising from the conventional view of the origins of the epidemic: that BSE arose from scrapie. At first, the use of the terms 'scrapie' and 'BSE' in the same sentence was not encouraged. Once the authorities realized that scrapie had never apparently spread to humans, the idea that BSE might be a form of scrapie suddenly became encouraged. Since people had remained unaffected by scrapie for centuries, it could be claimed that they would not catch BSE either. The fact that the infection could not jump that species barrier became a tenet of faith.

This does not stand up to examination. If scrapie were to be claimed as the origin of BSE, then a species jump from sheep to cattle must have occurred. If it could happen once, why not several times? For all the governmental proclamations encouraging people to forget about risks and to carry on eating beef and beef products, many biologists were speculating on the possibility that the next jump might be to *Homo sapiens* – the human species. To some, it was not a question of 'if', but 'when'. Although this alternative possibility has not been widely discussed, it may yet turn out that the BSE did *not* arise from scrapie. There are other possibilities, and we will return to them in Chapter 8.

Meanwhile, what of the risks? Government statements have insisted that beef is safe, and that there is no cause for public concern. That was a misrepresentation of the scientific position. The possibility of risks to people was ever-present in the published scientific conclusions, and the official insistence that there was nothing to worry about cannot be sustained. The reports suggested we should be watchful. They also proposed that any case of human spongy-brain disease contracted from infected beef would be similar to classical Creutzfeldt-Jakob disease. The Southwood report (see Chapter 8) in 1989 said this:

> 'It is a reasonable assumption that were BSE to be transmitted to humans, the clinical disorder would closely resemble CJD. Depending on the route of transmission, the incubation period could be as little as a year . . . or several decades.'

Birth of a New Disease?

In 1994 a strange new outbreak of spongy-brain disease did occur. It did resemble CJD, but there were a number of differences which indicated that this was something new.

- In Creutzfeldt-Jakob disease, forgetfulness is an early sign; in this new disease anxiety and uncharacteristic depression first appear.
- Victims of classical CJD typically succumb within six months, whilst in the new cases they survived for more than a year.
- The microscopical appearance of the new cases was distinct from what is seen in CJD.
- The average age for the onset of CJD is over sixty; in the new cases the average age was below thirty.

It was the youth of the new patients which was so disturbing. The first to be recorded was eighteen-year-old Victoria Rimmer of Connagh's Quay in North Wales. Vicky fell ill in 1994 and was still in a deep coma in hospital in early 1996. When thirty-year-old Maurice Callaghan died of spongy-brain disease in Belfast in

1995, his grave was dug nine feet deep, rather than six, and it is said that the gravediggers wore protective clothing and rubber gloves whilst dealing with his interment.

The relatives of these tragic victims most often claimed that infected beef was the likely cause. Victoria Rimmer's family always blamed the hamburgers she loved. When Jean Wake of Sunderland died at the age of thirty-eight, her children and her mother at her bedside, beef was blamed, too. She had worked in a pie factory, and her mother Mrs Nora Greenhalgh was convinced that infected beef had led to the death of her daughter. She added, 'I think that the reason people were kept in the dark was motivated by money.'

Last October Mrs Greenhalgh wrote to No. 10 Downing Street, to draw the attention of the Prime Minister to the possibility. The reply came from Ms Rachel Roberts, private secretary to the Prime Minister. It was quoted in *The Times*: 'I should make it clear that humans do not get "mad cow disease", although there are similar diseases which naturally occur in humans and have been known about for very many years,' she wrote. 'I must reassure you that there is no evidence to suggest that eating meat causes this sort of illness in people.'

These statements present a misleading impression. A year earlier, the official scientific view (see Chapter 8) had been this:

> ' . . . the BSE agent may be a human pathogen . . . it is too early to draw any conclusions because the incubation period in kuru, for example, can exceed thirty years.'

Mrs Greenhalgh did not believe what the Prime Minister's office was telling her. As we shall see, many of her doubts were shared by the scientific community. The population were closer to the view of scientists than the Government seemed to be.

In February 1996 a vegetarian student named Peter Hall, from Chester-le-Street in County Durham, died of the same condition. His vegetarian diet might make one look for different causes, but it turns out that he ate hamburgers as a youngster. His mother Frances sensibly believes that, if there were even a small chance of BSE being passed to people, official policies should always err on the side of safety. Peter Hall died just before his twenty-first birthday.

In Manchester, twenty-nine-year-old Michelle Brown died in November 1995 just three weeks after giving birth to her son Tony. Stephen Churchill, a promising student, died in May 1995 aged nineteen, after a year-long illness marked by dizziness and depression. Within a year there were over ten cases of this new form of spongy-brain disease known to the authorities.

Why was there no official response? There were plenty of people showing an interest in the subject. The topic is tailor-made for investigative journalists. An early writer on the scene was Peter Martin of the *Mail on Sunday*. His findings indicated that there were enough new cases to suggest that a new strain of spongy-brain disease was on the loose. Seven case histories had turned up in his investigations, with symptoms that seemed different from those of conventional Creutzfeldt-Jakob disease. He suggested that the new cases might be related to mad cow disease. The results were published in December 1995.

The Cannibals' Disease in the UK

The response of the Government to the report was immediate. The article was 'misleading and untrue', said Angela Browning, the Junior Minister for Agriculture.

The official view was obdurate; such stories were scaremongering.

Behind the scenes, however, the evidence was being collated. On 20 March 1996 the weight of data was too much to resist, and an official statement was made. The Secretary of State for Health, Stephen Dorrell, and the Secretary of State for Agriculture, Douglas Hogg, told the House of Commons that ten cases of a new form of spongy-brain disease were now known to the authorities. It was believed that BSE-infected beef might have been the culprit.

Once again, this was a classical example of unprofessional behaviour and poor timing. All we had was the government announcement in the House of Commons. There was no scientific paper to consult, no summary of the findings to guide enquirers. In science it is normal to publish results for everyone to see. Any official announcement can then be related to the facts. In this case the Government came out with its own version whilst the report was not yet available. Perhaps they hoped to look pro-active and direct. It is possible they sought to defuse the impact of the paper by starting an informal debate before it was available.

The papers on these tragic cases had been prepared and were already being printed. They were published on 5 April 1996 in the medical journal the *Lancet*, 347: 921–948. The microscopical examination of brain sections from these cases showed an appearance rather different from that of Creutzfeldt-Jakob disease, CJD. Officially, it was announced that a new strain of CJD had been discovered.

I do not believe that is a tenable conclusion. A 'new strain' of disease is classified as being a subdivision of the illness which it most resembles. The appearance of the brain sections were different from classical CJD, and closer to those of scrapie. They were just like those from victims of the cannibal disease from Papua New Guinea. The bizarre behaviour of the victims was exactly like that described since the 1950s in the Fore tribe. There is only one conclusion I can draw: these young Britons have died of kuru. It was more than anyone could admit.

The dramatic announcement had all the wrong results. The British authorities were panicked into announcing a range of ill-thought-out measures. The European Union responded by imposing a worldwide ban on British beef products, so that Cadbury's even had to halt the export of their Curly Wurly chocolates. The world's press was on our doorstep, yet the Government had little to show them. How limited is their understanding of the science which governs our lives.

Confidence in the honesty of government has long been declining. Now, at a stroke, the authorities alienated scientists, too. Overnight, the beef industry was disrupted, and everyone in the land felt that sense of disillusionment, even panic.

Public suspicions had been right all along. The Government had been wrong.

6

WHERE'S THE BEEF?

One thing used to bother me as a child interested in anatomy. I remember reading the anatomy texts, and wondering where the meat might be. In all the diagrams there was plenty of bone, impressive areas of skin, endless organs and litres of blood, but – not a sign of anything labelled 'meat'.

Meat is muscle. The body is controlled by the intricate network of muscles that provide our posture and maintain our movement. The white meat from a crab's claws, or from the tail of scampi or lobster, is the massive muscle which the animal uses to eat and to move. It's the main muscle which is eaten in shrimps and prawns, cockles and mussels. The breast of chicken is the main flight muscle, the largest in the body of birds, whilst rump steak comes from the rear end of cattle – the largest muscle mass in mammals.

Different nations use a carcase in different ways. British butchers tend to slice meat in hunks, irrespective of the detailed anatomy, whereas French butchers tend more to follow the anatomy of an animal and consider each muscle as a structure on its own. There are tremendous food fads, of course: dogs and snakes are a delicacy in many parts of the world and horsemeat is enjoyed in much of Europe. We will examine some of these shades of opinion a little later (Chapter 9). In Britain we eat a lot of lamb; it is less often found in Europe and is regarded as a rare fad in the USA.

Consumption of chicken (a luxury a few decades ago) has greatly increased since intensive rearing became available, and new presentations of food are always sought by purchasers. Nutritionists have taught that people eat what their parents ate, which is a nonsensical view. If it were true there would be no pizzas or lasagne, no satay sauce or balsamic vinegar. Indian and Chinese restaurants would never have become so popular in Britain, and the hamburger would remain an American oddity.

Our liking for food depends on what our peers like. It is influenced by fashions, which rise and fall from time to time, and by the power of advertising. Behind it all lurks a fondness for tradition. The taste of roast beef and Yorkshire pudding, for many people, is a link with security. The roast joint was associated with traditional family meals. Even in an age when relatively few people roast meat at home, the favourite choice for Sunday lunch at a pub or restaurant is still a roast. Set down a dotted line followed by the words '... of olde England' and most would fill in 'roast beef'.

What's in a Steak?

The best beef for many people is the fillet. This is a rather small muscle near the kidneys and inside the ribcage, so it is tender and soft. It is relatively free of fibrous tissue. Cheaper cuts come from the muscles of the limbs, and they are often made into minced meat or sold as brisket.

Excess fat, together with offcuts, are made into sausages and pies, savoury duck, haslet (sometimes called acelet) or faggots. Bull calves produce more meat than cows; three-quarters (75 per cent) of a bull is lean meat, compared with two-thirds (66 per cent) of a cow.

Once the lean meat has been removed, the rest of the carcase has many uses. The hide may well be tanned and made into leather goods. The bones are sometimes cooked for sale as pet food, or made into meal. This is sometimes used as animal feed and also as a garden fertilizer. What can't be utilized is rendered down for the extraction of gelatine. The blood is collected and used to make black pudding – a highly nutritious, if fattening, food – or it may be dried for use as a fertilizer. Sub-standard animals go to make pet foods, and so do inedible portions of healthy carcases.

Once all the usable meat has been removed, the remaining portions of the carcase still contain edible animal protein. This is then processed to provide mechanically recovered meat. Traces of meat are stripped from hides and bones, and the remainder is crushed to squeeze out any that remains. There is much emotional comment on processes like these, but there is nothing inherently less aesthetic about eating one sort of animal tissue if you readily eat another. In principle, the only differences are appearance – and safety. Mechanically recovered meat is unappetizing and pasty. It has high nutriment value, of course, and has long been considered an acceptable additive to cheap pies, frozen burger products and pâtés.

Beef By-products

The cattle-farming industry provides us with an incredibly long list of products:

- Main cuts: include rump and fillet, sirloin and silverside. Fore and prime ribs, topside, flank and skirt are cheaper cuts.
- Hide and tendons: the main use of animal skin is leather and vellum. This ancient form of paper is produced from thin layers of animal hide, and is still used for the production of ceremonial documents and book conservation.
- Unusable hide (along with tendons, ligaments, cartilage and bones) is rendered down to produce gelatine.
- Bones: sold as pet food, garden fertilizer, bone-meal, and also to make bone stock for use in gravies (including 'chicken' and 'lamb' gravy products).
- Mechanically recovered meat: this product, MRM for short, goes to supplement pies and hamburgers, soups and stews, sausages and pâtés.
- Vertebrae are banned for extraction of MRM, but are used for other bone products.
- Beef extract: sold in jars as Bovril, and also included in many sausage products including peperoni and frankfurters. Up to 20 per cent of pork sausages can comprise beef products.
- Milk: sold as the daily pint on the British doorstep (now a diminishing business), and used to make sterilized and UHT products, skimmed milk, cream, cheese, whey, yoghurt; an ingredient of many other products from chocolate to soup.
- Lactose: one of the sugars, a relative of the sweet sucrose which is the sugar in the sugar-bowl, lactose has many uses as a filler and as a flavour-carrier in products like crisps
- Fat: a source of tallow with many industrial applications (including the manufacture of soap and candles). Beef fat also goes to make dripping and lard, and is found in lamb and chicken stews. The granular fat sold as suet is widely used in catering.
- Glycerol: a major by-product of beef fat, glycerol is found in many medicines and foods. Its syrupy texture and sweetish taste give it many uses in cookery.
- Elastin: many cosmetic products use beef by-products, and

elastin is extracted from waste carcase matter. It is the elastic component of fibrous tissues in animals.

- Keratin: this protein product makes up horns, hair and hooves. Keratin is a popular ingredient of 'repair' shampoos.
- Oleo oil: made from beef fat and a common ingredient of butter-like food products
- Stearic acid and stearin: these important products are used to make soaps and sweets, waterproofing and candles, metal polish and cosmetics. Stearates are found in body-building supplements.
- Rennet: contains an enzyme, rennin, which clots the protein in milk. It is used to make junket, and is important in the first stages of cheese manufacture when the curds are separated from the whey.

As can be seen, the range of products is extensive and their uses are extremely wide. Vegetarians and vegans are posed particular problems by this diversification. Vegetarians are officially defined by the Vegetarian Society as persons who do not eat any meat, fowl, fish or other seafood, nor any of their by-products. In practice many vegetarians have habits that are rather more lax than this strict definition. Though they confine themselves (mostly) to eating vegetable products, many of them also eat fish. Some consume white meat, like chicken breast, whilst others eat curries which contain a little meat.

The Vegan Culture

Vegans are far more strict than vegetarians. The Vegan Society say they prohibit the eating of any product from animal sources, and they include eggs, animal milk, cheese and yoghurt, honey and all of their derivatives. Sometimes this compassionate view can perhaps go too far. I have heard of one young mother who was ostracized by a vegan group because she was breast-feeding her baby. Milk of animal origins is banned, and her natural behaviour towards her newborn child incurred the wholesale disapproval of her friends. My response was to say that the aim of vegetarian and vegan diets is to alleviate any suffering or unwitting exploitation of animals. In this case the child was naturally exploiting the mother (all babies act as parasites, a trend which can be unnaturally prolonged in modern society) but she was blameless. The misuse of well-meaning practices as sanctions against one's fellows is a regrettable facet of human life.

One rare book on the subject published in Cornwall has the intriguing title *The Bible, black pudding, mad-cow disease, and the human sexuality report*. It was published in the form of typewritten pages. The author, Ronald Dinner, argues that abstinence from black pudding would cut your chances of contracting mad cow disease. 'It stands to reason that eating flesh is more likely to transmit diseases than eating fruit, vegetables and cereal foods,' he says. This has a certain self-evident clarity about it, but it is not true. It's certainly clear that animal foods are more likely to transmit animal *infections*, but *diseases* are a different matter. Many of the problems from mutations and cancers are more easily related to the vegetables in our diet. This is perhaps the most idiosyncratic book containing advice about the spongiform encephalopathies. Its subtitle explains that the book is a response to: 'Why Bible-believing Methodists shouldn't eat black pudding and the "Human sexuality report", at the Methodist Conference of 1993'.

Diets of vegetables can be dangerous. High levels of fibre are associated with gut problems. Many plants contain carcinogenic and mutagenic compounds which can damage DNA, and pulses can contain a long list of potentially hazardous components. Food-poisoning bacteria can lurk on the skin of uncooked fruit and vegetables, and the high proportion of water in such foods can result in lowered levels of nutriment.

Devoted vegetarians and vegans take care to balance their diet in order to ensure that a full range of vitamins and amino acids is consumed. You cannot eat safely by merely leaving out the meat if you have always enjoyed a traditionally omnivorous diet in the past. There is a claim that the word vegetarian derives from a Latin word *vegetus* meaning 'lively'. It's true that there was a word 'vegete', which died out earlier in the century, and it was defined by the *Oxford English Dictionary* as 'healthy and active; flourishing in respect of health and vigour'. However, the introduction of the term vegetarian in the 1840s seems to have referred to vegetables rather than vitality.

A diet of vegetables is not a natural diet. The human species is clearly intended to be omnivorous. There are many reasons why this is so, and human anatomy provides the evidence.

	Herbivores	Carnivores	Humans
Eyes	On side of head	Front of head	Front of head
Appendix	Very large	Absent	Very small
Base of tooth	Large hole	No hole	Small hole
Crown of tooth	Flat and worn	Irregular	Fairly smooth
Canine tooth	Missing	Prominent	Present

Table 6: Characteristics of Carnivores and Herbivores

On the basis of anatomy, there can be no real question that mankind evolved as an omnivorous species. The canine tooth and the position of the eyes suggests that, if there is a predisposition one way or the other, then the carnivorous option is somewhat dominant.

Many non-meat-eaters base their feelings, not on such scientific considerations, but on compassionate or humanitarian grounds. They do not approve of modern agricultural methods and seek to show their feelings by refusing to support intensive farming that may be insufficiently considerate of the well-being of farm animals. Few people can argue with the sincerity of that. Intensive farming with an eye on the bottom line is what gave rise to the practices which seem to have resulted in BSE. Compassionate farming is a timely and constructive concept.

Some people change to vegetarianism by cutting down on red meat, then on white, and eventually they give up fish as well. They decline to eat meat because they are no longer used to it. They don't like the taste, and find the texture unpleasant. There has been a long-term trend away from eating beef in Britain. In 1980 the average amount consumed was 20 kg per person; currently it is just over 15 kg per head, a drop of a quarter in sixteen years.

Giving up Meat

It is far harder to give up meat products than you might imagine. There is, surprisingly, no beef at all in beef-flavoured crisps and snack products. There isn't any in Bisto powder, nor in Marmite. At least one proprietary brand of steak pie contains no beef whatever. On the other hand, there are beef products in wine gums and liquorice allsorts, in marshmallows and ice-cream. There is British beef (or its by-products) in wholemeal digestive biscuits, most pork sausages, mincemeat and pork pies.

British beef products	Foreign beef products	No beef products
Liquorice allsorts	Wine gums	Roast beef crisps
Fruit fool puddings	Fromage frais	Bisto powder
Christmas pudding	Turkish delight	Marmite
Sweet mincemeat	Chocolate finger biscuits	Campbell's meatballs
Pork pies	Pork pâté	Wall's pork sausages
Wholewheat biscuits	Marshmallows	Ginsters sausage rolls
Oxo cubes	Stock cubes	McCain pizzas
Rowntree's jelly	Paxo stuffing	Fish paste

Table 7: Beef Products in Everyday Foods

These many uses make a truly vegan lifestyle a matter of single-minded determination. There are beef products in the most unexpected places. Interestingly, in many of the products where you would expect to find a lot of beef it is less in evidence. The proportion of beef in beef pies can be surprisingly small, especially when you bear in mind that half of the modest beef content may be in the form of mechanically recovered meat or beef fat. There are many beef-flavoured snacks and crisps on sale, and none of the examples I have seen contain any beef at all.

Are by-products of beef a danger to health? Time will tell, but the current claims are that this is unlikely. In many cases the beef product is gelatine, and this is made by heating bones, hide and other animal waste products under pressure. The proportion of nervous tissue is small, and it is hoped that the conditions under which the gelatine is produced might inactivate the agent of BSE. I am not aware of experiments to prove the point. Until we know, the banning of gelatine from British beef carcases does make sense. In this area, too, we need more data than are currently available.

Meat and meat products have long been an essential component of Western life. Quite apart from the prehistoric leather industry, even such familiar products as candles from beef tallow remind us that we have been using cattle as a source of raw materials since before recorded time. The widespread application of beef products is nothing new, and it is not solely a result of modern technology.

Safety, however, is another matter. Never before have we seen the outbreak of such a potentially serious medical problem, and until BSE has been effectively controlled we may have to look again at many processes we have believed to be safe for centuries.

7

REAL COWS ARE CARNIVORES

The first cattle came to Europe with the neolithic people some 30,000 years ago. In recorded history, beef was for many centuries a food only for the ruling class. After the Norman Conquest, their Anglo-Saxon subjects, through to the end of the thirteenth century, looked enviously at the noblemen who alone could afford such luxury. That is why roast beef has remained a special meal. It is not something you expect to find served in the middle of the week. Beef was traditionally reserved for Sundays.

There is one cow for every four people in the world. The largest population of cattle is in China, where there are over 600 million. There are 100 million cattle in the USA, 125 million in Europe, and 12 million in Britain. The quality of the cow varies considerably. In Europe we expect a carcase weight of about 250 kg, whilst in China it is only 75 kg, and is 80 kg in India. The United States sets the world record with an average carcase weight of 271 kg, with Britain a little behind at 260 kg.

Few people outside the farming world know much of how cattle are reared. There are several methods in use, depending on the fertility of the farm and the end-product.

- Beef from spring-born steers on fertile farms are typically produced on a cycle that begins in February. Male calves are bought and, at the same time, finished cattle are sold. In April the year-old castrated cattle are put out to graze, and may also be fed on concentrates. These supplements, along with home-grown silage, are often what help to sustain the animals during the winter. Under ideal circumstances a growing calf can put on weight at the rate of almost 1 kg per day. After two years, the heaviest cattle will weigh about 680 kg, 380 kg when slaughtered and dressed. This provides 270 kg lean meat, 60 kg bone and 50 kg trimmed fat.
- Suckler beef can be produced on more marginal land. A 'cow unit' comprises a cow, a calf and a yearling. Calving takes place between February and April, and the young animals grow rapidly on their diet of mother's milk. The yearlings are allowed to eat as much silage as they wish, with an additional 1 kg of concentrates per day. This system gives a final weight at 20 months of 500-600 kg, with a dressed carcase weight between 250-330 kg.
- The most productive form of beef is from bull calves. They grow up to 8 per cent faster than the heifers and produce carcases that are 15 per cent heavier. They also produce a higher proportion of premium cuts, so they are more profitable to raise. Bull beef is not of the highest quality, and the *cognoscenti* tend to avoid it. Young bulls are raised on a diet which may be home-made, or contain concentrates, meal and roughage. They can put on weight at 1-1.4 kg per day and are ready for slaughter at 12 months. Bulls are raised in pens which provide 2-5 square metres of space per animal, with up to 25 bulls in each pen. They are strong and powerful animals, and raising them demands care for the farm-workers' personal safety.

The humane treatment of cattle is required by international law. There are fixed conditions of transportation and rest, or feeding and watering. It is tempting to assume that nobody takes much notice, but there are strong financial incentives which encourage dealers to handle cattle sympathetically. Stress produces poor quality beef of a dark and dry texture. Only when animals are relaxed and well-watered are they fit to make the best price for the seller. Greed is no incentive to cruelty in this situation.

Slaughter

Cattle are taken to slaughter and are shot through the forehead with a captive bolt gun. This is a pistol in which the bullet does not separate from the weapon, but takes the form of a captive bolt which shoots out a few inches and can be set again for re-use. The stunned beast is then hung up and bled. If this is not done properly, the resulting meat will be suffused and blotchy. Halal slaughter is favoured by Islamic traditions and dispatches an animal by a single cut across the throat, but without any prior stunning.

The beef carcase has head and hooves removed. Both the gullet and rectum are tied so that the entire digestive tract can be discarded, and the offal (the internal organs) are removed and put on conveyors. All parts are supposed to be inspected by qualified veterinarians. Then the carcase is flayed (skinned) and split down the middle. The spinal cord is removed and discarded, with varying degrees of effectiveness. Both sides are weighed and inspected, and on this basis the payment is made – usually on the basis of warm weight minus 2 per cent to cover the weight lost by evaporation as the meat cools. The sides are then washed and hung in a room to cool.

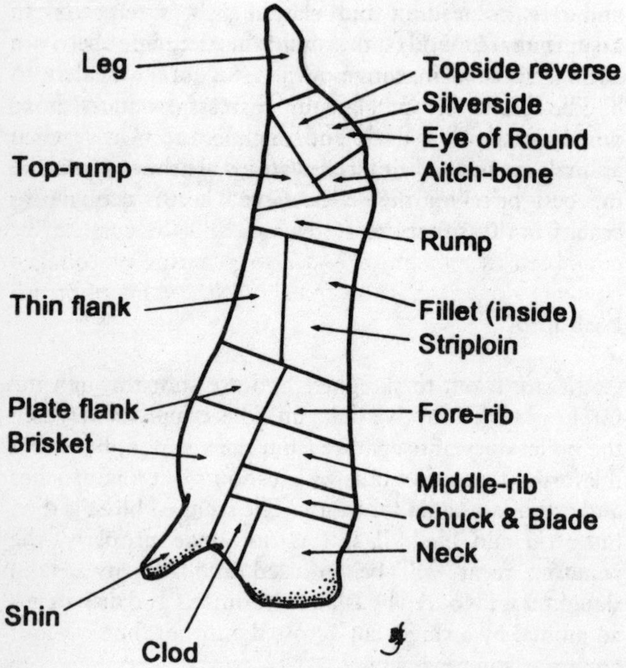

Fig 4: Cuts of Beef

After slaughter the beef carcase is cut into portions that have traditional names. The exact method of cutting varies from one country to another, and even from region to region. Fillet, a muscle near the kidneys from inside the carcase, is the most tender steak of all. Other cuts (like skirt or skirting, from the ribs) are tender, too.

The cooling process has to be gradual; if meat is cooled below 10°C within ten hours, it will toughen and lose value. Before it is cut, beef should be below 7°C. It can take thirty-six hours to reach this temperature in a cooling room at freezing-point.

There is much debate, amongst steak-eaters, as to which cut is most tender. The toughness of meat depends on the amount of collagen it contains. The more collagen in a cut, the more tough is the meat. There is a toughness scale from 0 (tough) to 8 (tender), and the cuts can be compared in tenderness and also in terms of collagen content. These results are typical for the quality of British beef:

Cut	Per cent collagen	Tenderness (0-8)
Fillet	2.2	6.5
Striploin	2.8	5.2
Rump	3.6	4.5
Topside	4.0	3.3
Eye of round	4.7	3.5
Silverside	5.0	2.8

Table 8: How tough is your beef-steak?

How Dangerous is Beef ?

There have been many reasons why people should cut down on the amount of beef they eat. Saturated fat is one major problem. The levels of fats in a Western diet are too high, and much of it comes from meat. Cutting back on beef consumption has been advised for that reason. Food poisoning is another. Some strains of *Salmonella* are particularly difficult to treat, and some of them are transmitted by hamburgers. There are carcinogens (chemicals capable of causing cancer) in charred and braised foods, and levels of these substances in the charcoal-grilled surface of steaks and burgers are relatively high. People have been warned of dangers from eating beef for years.

The new problems from BSE are impossible to quantify. However, it is believed that it is the central nervous system (brain and spinal cord) which poses the greatest hazard, and if that is the case then the regular cuts of beef are currently construed as relatively safe.

The Milk Business

One of the earliest areas of concern was over the safety of milk, and about this we have relatively little evidence to go on. Almost all our milk comes from cows. There is a growing market for soya milk, a substitute made with protein and fat from soy beans. Goat's milk has a following amongst health-food fanatics. It is unlikely to produce the allergies associated with cow's milk, which is good news. But goat farming is not as well regulated as are cattle, and the problems of contamination are likely to be higher for that reason alone.

Of the twelve million cattle in Britain, less than three million produce milk. The average cow produces about 5,400 litres of milk per year. That's an annual British total of fourteen billion litres. Cows produce milk after giving birth to their young, and they produce their first calves when they are two years old. For the first four days after giving birth the cow produces colostrum. Colostrum passes many useful substances to the calf (antibodies against disease, for instance) and is not suitable for human consumption. From the fifth day onwards, the cow produces milk and this is what the farmer hopes to sell for profit. If there is no further pregnancy, the cow produces milk for ten months after calving. Three months after giving birth she can be made pregnant again. This pregnancy lasts for nine months, for the last two of which the cow does not produce milk. Cows are capable of up to ten periods of lactation during their lives, though the national average is below five. They are then slaughtered at six to seven years. Cows would otherwise live for fifteen years or more.

One frequently asked question is : why does a cow produce milk? It's a sensible enquiry. Other adult mammals don't, unless they happen to be feeding their young. The trick is to remove the calf when just a day or two old, and then to keep milking. The removal of milk from the cow acts as a stimulus for the glands to produce more milk. It works, too. Most dairy farmers milk their cows twice a day. Some have tried milking three times daily instead, and their cows produce up to 15 per cent more milk.

The topic one never hears about is the day when the calves are taken from their mothers. Cows are affectionate and loyal. They are protective towards their young. On the day that the truck comes to collect the calves, a sad and mournful wailing goes up from the deprived mothers. Most farm-workers hate the day when the calves are collected. This pitiful spectacle is rarely mentioned outside farming circles, and is never in the minds of those city-dwellers who regard milk as the most natural food on earth.

Milk is far from being 'natural', unless you happen to be a calf.

Is Milk Safe?

Unpasteurized milk can transmit tuberculosis, brucellosis and other conditions. They are relatively rare, however.

Far more common is the fact that many people are allergic to milk and to dairy products in general. For them, milk in the diet is a hazard to health. Lactose intolerance is found in a significant number of people, and the lactose in milk is an additional problem for them.

The original recommendation was that milk from cows with BSE should be discarded. Though it is hard to disagree with the sense of that advice, it would have made more sense had we decided to maintain an approach based on the immediate elimination of all BSE-infected cattle. The agent of BSE has not been found in milk, and the proportion of calves contracting BSE does not suggest that they got it from milk.

There are some advantages in unpasteurized raw milk. It has a special taste which you can only expect to find on a farm. For many years the sale of unpasteurized milk was unlawful, but now it can be sold with the following government warning:

> 'This milk has not been treated and therefore may contain organisms harmful to your health'.

It is also rich in enzymes and other components which heat treatment destroys. Many people swear by it. Organic milk is a different matter. This has to conform to specified practices:

- Calves must be fed on organic milk from their natural or foster mother, or from the bucket, until they are at least nine weeks old.
- Cattle must not be fed any animal matter (such as meat and bone-meal).
- Sixty per cent of their diet must be hay, silage or grass
- Antibiotics are not to be used except to treat a specific illness.
- Any milk containing traces of antibiotics is not to be sold for consumption.

One enduring problem for all farmers is the complex system of levies and rewards imposed by Brussels under the Common Agricultural Policy or CAP. I have yet to speak to a farmer who privately approves of the system. Farming is the biggest business in Britain, and farmers are traditionally Conservative voters, which might explain why government has been unwilling to find ways to cut these liberal subsidies.

The fact that farming is all controlled by decree makes nonsense of a 'free market' economy. Currently, farmers receive 25p per litre for their milk. The amount they can produce is limited by quota, and if a dairy farm produces more than this limit it is fined more than 30p per litre. Many farmers throw away their surplus milk, when they would rather it went to fulfil a social need – perhaps by distribution to hospitals, for example.

When the dairy industry does change, it is not necessarily because of demands imposed by economics. Fashions and fads dictate what farmers will produce, and the consumer can always have the upper hand. A generation ago, skimmed milk was a waste product. It was what remained after cream had been separated off. The increasing emphasis on a fat-free diet has made skimmed and semi-skimmed milk into popular products which now outsell whole milk. As a result, the by-product, cream, is being produced in larger amounts than can be consumed. It has to go somewhere, so cream is added to an increasingly wide range of food products. As consumers prefer to add fashionable skimmed milk to their tea they may save a few grams of fat intake per day. But then they have a vegetable soup from a can at lunchtime, and that contains the very cream which they would have had in the morning milk.

It is the young female calves, the heifers, which can be raised for milk production. The male calves are usually sold on for later sale as veal at the age of about six months. In Britain, a bull calf is worth only some £20, but if it is sold for veal production in Europe the value rises to £150. Half a million veal calves are therefore exported every year. Live exports are widely disliked in modern Britain, and one can easily see why this is. The fact is that agricultural practices vary widely in countries separated by a few miles of water (yet, nominally, intimately joined in the European Union) and this is what needs to change. To tell a farmer that he should not export a bull calf out of principle is all very well, but if it costs him £130 each time he agrees it imposes an unfair disadvantage on his business.

Such matters could easily brought into common practice throughout Europe. Like the fact that the duty on alcoholic drinks is ten times higher in Britain than on the mainland of Europe, this is an area where Brussels could usefully intervene. Perhaps interference in flavoured crisps or sausages could come after these more pressing matters were solved.

Keeping Cattle

The most fundamental issue of all is how we keep cattle in captivity. How do we ensure that the conditions match the natural needs of the cows? There was a fascinating forecast made more than seventy years ago, which seemed to predict our present predicament. The occasion was a lecture in the Swiss town of Dornach, and the speaker was a philosopher and advocate of natural farming named Rudolf Steiner. It was 1923.

'If an ox were to eat meat directly, it would go crazy,' he said. The outbreak of BSE seems to make this a prophecy come true – or does it? Steiner was guessing, using empty claims to advance his views. The making of groundless threats is a common occurrence, and it is always an easy temptation to look back at some rambling comment and regard it as a prediction. The difference between a guess and a real prediction lies in the reasoned basis for the proposal. Rudolf Steiner had some clear ideas on natural organic farming (they were obvious ideas, but they did make some sense) but many of his other views were most peculiar. He held a theory that acids build up in the system if there is unused energy in the body, and he seems to have understood remarkably little about real physiology or current scientific knowledge.

The idea of a cannibal cow is clearly disturbing, put baldly, but to make a wild prognostication on little real evidence does not, in my view, amount to a prediction of the future. To what extent is the diet of today's cattle 'cannibalistic'? There are clear resonances between the idea of feeding animal products to cattle and the eating of the brains of the deceased amongst the Fore people of Papua New Guinea. To some people there is a moral lesson here, as though nature were punishing us for cutting corners. They feel that something unnatural must be avoided at all costs.

The notion of 'naturalness' is seductive, but being civilized is a highly unnatural state and we need unnatural means to survive. However, as we create new approaches to old problems it is always important try to fit our new strategies to be sympathetic to the way life used to be. We cannot throw over tried and tested traditions without careful consideration.

How Cows are Carnivorous

Cows are natural carnivores. They have never lived on grass. Cows cannot digest plant tissues. My seemingly heretical view needs explanation, so let us travel down

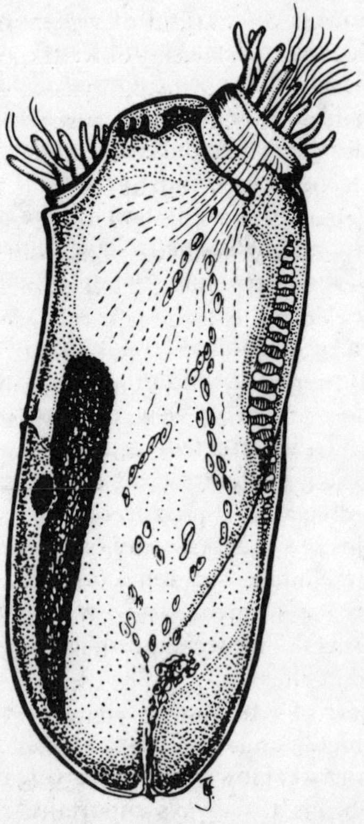

Fig 5: *Epidinium*

The rumen of cows (a false stomach) is really a fermentation reactor in which grass collected by the animal becomes the diet of teeming communities of microbes. The largest microbes are animal cells, protozoa, like this beautiful Epidinium. *These microbes, which can just be seen with the naked eye, are then digested by the cow.*

a cow's gullet with its food and observe what happens. The cow takes a mouthful of vegetation and chews it. The mashed mass slips easily down the gullet, but it never reaches the stomach. Instead, it passes into the *rumen,* a chambered pouch filled with a semi-solid, fermenting mass.

The rumen comes above the stomach. It is formed from an expansion of the lower end of the gullet itself. Inside it lives a teeming community of microbes. Many of them are bacteria, but the top of the food chain are protozoa. They are single-celled animal organisms, the largest of which are just visible to the naked eye. This community of tiny cells can digest the grass, because the microbes secrete enzymes which break down the cell walls of the vegetable diet on which the cow subsists.

In order to mix the mass, to help break down the dissolving vegetation, and to ensure there is plenty of oxygen in the brew, the cow repeatedly regurgitates the rumen contents and chews it, over and over again. As we have seen, the phenomenon of rumination is characteristic of all these animals. In time, the plant matter has been digested by the microbes which have multiplied in the process. This is how the plant protein on which the cow grazed is converted into protozoan protein – animal matter. It is animal protein, and not grass, which passes into the cow's stomach and intestines where conventional digestion takes place.

Thus, cattle have always existed by digesting animal protein. Feeding them meal containing the right sort of animal matter is not self-evidently inappropriate. On its own, there is nothing to suggest that this process causes disease. It is not new. Cows have always digested animal protein, and there is no reason why the wise use of safe and germ-free supplements should not play its part in farming for a new millennium.

8

FOOD FRIGHT

Food scares have always featured in society. Every few years, sometimes every few months, there is some frightening new disclosure about our diet. Earlier in the twentieth century there were fears that the influence of electrical wiring could threaten people's health, and many cooks said they would prefer to prepare meals on a range in the traditional manner. The contemporary counterpart to their concerns are the questions now being asked about high-tension cables and electricity pylons.

By the 1920s aluminium cooking pots and pans were the target of attack, and many kitchens turned their backs on these new additions to the range. The objections were soon laughed to scorn, though there has been a revival of interest in the possible health hazards of aluminium in recent years. Some research has suggested that raised levels of aluminium are found in the brains of people who have died of Alzheimer's disease. There's no evidence that it is the cause.

In the 1970s the target of disapproval was potatoes. Women who had eaten meals made with traces of still-green potatoes were told their unborn children might be at risk.

When Fads are Useful

Food scares aren't always bad news. There have been cases where one has been useful. For instance, spina bifida, which baffled medicine for centuries, has been shown to be related to low levels of folate in the diet, and supplements of this kind are now believed to help ward off this tragically disabling condition.

In some instances, fads undergo a polarizing change of opinion. In the 1960s, the foods you were supposed to avoid if you wished to go on a diet were bread and potatoes. Twenty-five years later, the recommendation for any conscientious dieter was to eat plenty of potatoes and bread. Sometimes it is hard to keep up with the latest trend.

Occasionally the dangers from diet are very real. An extreme allergy to walnuts can kill susceptible people. Peanuts, a common constituent of modern foods, are often contaminated with aflatoxins which are known to cause genetic mutations. The sensitization of a person with a very small dose of some foods can make them hypersensitive to future exposure, sometimes with fatal consequences. In the summer of 1996 there is an example of this. Increasing numbers of children have been reported with a peanut allergy. One survey suggests that there may be 65,000 British children in this category; one child became unwell when a packet of peanuts was opened across the room.

Another food scare for the summer of 1996 is a new threat of tuberculosis from pigs. Birds have been found to pass on a *Mycobacterium* infection through their droppings. Whether this bacterium will present a hazard to humans remains to be seen, and the extent to which this may be a real health problem is uncertain. There are, then, several current new controversies over our food.

War Against Meat

Meat has often been a target for attack. One of the most ancient prohibitions applies, not to beef, but to pork. The Semitic races, Arabs and Jews among others, still proscribe the eating of pork and pork products. The ancient teachings clearly recognized the transmission to people of a parasitic worm, *Trichinella spiralis*, which forms cysts through the muscles and causes generalized weakness and disease. Modern farming methods have eliminated *Trichinella* in Europe, and the worm is in any event killed by the normal temperatures used in cooking.

It is in America that the greatest scare campaigns have been waged against meat. Beef was condemned by Sylvester Graham's fervent campaigning, along with any cooked vegetables. Jerome Irvine weighed in against wheat, sugar and anything cooked. One leading proponent of a meat-free diet was William Kellogg, who went on to found the great cereal company.

Meat has been associated with a raised cancer risk, and barbecued beef in particular contains benzpyrenes (a known cancer-causing complex). Meat is served with salt, and that is now associated with an increased risk of high blood pressure in susceptible individuals. In the last year a new strain of food-poisoning germ has been identified in hamburgers. It is said to cause severe illness and is unusually difficult to treat.

The fat component of beef, as we have seen, is a further hazard:

- Firstly, it adds to the calories in the diet.
- Second, fats decompose quickly and produce chemicals which damage DNA and cause mutations.
- Third, saturated fats (the kind found in beef) are associated with coronary heart disease.

People have been warned against eating beef (or, at least, eating too much beef) for generations. Many of these health hazards seem to pose a greater risk of disease than the evidence so far laid against beef transmitting BSE to humans.

Enter a New Disease

Few scientists were surprised to learn that there might be a new strain of CJD (Creutzfeldt-Jakob disease, the human equivalent of mad cow disease). The fact that the victims have been younger, and that the course of their illness has been different from typical CJD, is what makes me conclude that we should not call it a strain of CJD at all. I am sure we are witnessing the re-emergence of a kind of kuru. If it needs a new name, then Human Spongiform Encephalopathy (HSE) might be the most suitable designation since we already have Feline Spongiform Encephalopathy (FSE) in cats.

What grounds are there for assuming that the new strain of spongy-brain disease came from cattle? There isn't any firm evidence that this new form arose from eating BSE-infected products, though it's a reasonable guess it might. BSE is a dramatic disease. It damages the brain. It is highly photogenic. The situation is a classical case, and was always bound to attract maximum attention.

The Government are the target for attack on all sides. They should have known better. They should have done more. We should never have believed them . . . yet how often do we stop to reflect on the impossible situation a government faces when there is a new threat like this? The way of politics is to set down principles in black and white: 'Is the Minister aware? Yes or no?' – we watch it each night in parliamentary reports, and hear these demands every morning on the radio. Admitting that an opinion may have been wrong, or having the grace to change your mind, can be a resigning matter in Parliament.

Scientific issues cannot be measured in terms like those. In BSE the unknowns are intriguing, and the science remains vague. You often hear of the 'virus' of mad cow disease. There isn't one. The cause of BSE is still a mystery. Viruses contain DNA or RNA, and the agent of BSE contains neither. We have seen that it survives cooking. It is not even attacked by normal disinfectants, and you need to expose it to highly dangerous solutions of chlorine bleach to inactivate it. Scientists have been asked to give advice on what to do – but science simply does not know the truth.

Prions

In sections of diseased tissue under the electron microscope we can see fine threads called *prions*. We do not know what they are there for. Indeed, although it's comforting to assume that the prion causes the illness, we can't even be certain of that. Maybe the misshapen prions form as a result of the disease. They could be a consequence, and not the cause.

In most infections, animals manifest the disease throughout the body. Evidence suggested that BSE might be confined to the central nervous system, so the Government made slaughterhouses remove the main nerves from

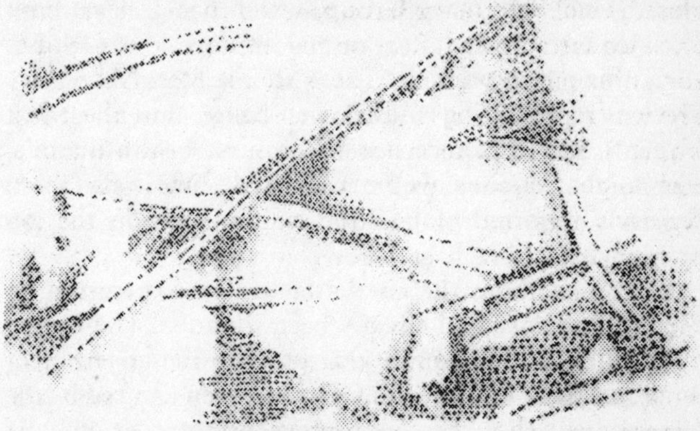

Fig 6: Prions

Under the high-power electron microscope, the ghostly images of long fibres can be seen in specimens from victims of spongy-brain diseases. These are the prions. They are not destroyed by cooking, and can resist most disinfectants. It may be that these are the infective agents which transmit the disease.

infected carcases, and stain them so that they could not be used in food. But this is the era when businessmen try to minimize their costs. Dyes cost money. So does the time to do the work, and so do senior slaughterhouse staff. It follows that cheap labour is often used, so there is nobody around to ensure the task is undertaken properly. The removal of offal is often done hastily, to save time and money. And I am still not aware of any way of ensuring that none of the condemned by-products end up in cheap mass-produced burgers, sausages and pies. Indeed, I cannot even imagine how such a system could be made to work in an era hungry for money at any cost.

The maintenance of standards in the industry is the responsibility of MAFF (the Ministry for Agriculture, Fisheries and Food). They have a panel, the Animal

Health and Veterinary Group, which has a clear remit to safeguard health and animal welfare. Two bodies carry this out in practice. These are the State Veterinary Service, representing animal well-being, and the Meat Hygiene Service, concerned with public health matters. The system sounds well-constructed, but it has been regularly reported to be short of funds to do the job properly.

Warnings about the risks attached to cost-cutting in the beef industry had already been sounded. The British Veterinary Association, a year prior to the government announcement on BSE and CJD, had been assured by the Government that these organizations were being fully supported. The BVA were not impressed. They went so far as to issue a document which specifically warned of the way matters were moving. Nobody could doubt the strong sense of their statement:

> 'It is clear that the proposals [in MAFF's review of the Animal Health and Veterinary Group] have very little to do with the . . . remit, namely safeguarding animal health and improving animal welfare, but have everything to do with cutting costs. There must be no short cuts with animal health, animal welfare or public health.'

Danger in the Abattoirs

A random sample of slaughterhouses was undertaken in 1995, and in the sample almost half the establishments (48 per cent) were failing in their handling of offal. In the knackers' yards only a third were doing the job properly, for they had a failure rate of 65 per cent. Since the controls were implemented there have been several attempts to tighten the regulations. Passing new regulations is much easier than making sure they are ever observed.

Sitting in the centre of the controversy have been the Government and their advisers. Until that fateful day in March 1996, when the House of Commons were told of the sudden outbreak of spongy-brain disease in the young, the official view had been simply expressed:

- British beef is perfectly safe.
- We have to go on what the scientists tell us.
- Scientists say that there is no evidence of any link between CJD and BSE.
- Standards of meat hygiene and safety are higher in Britain than anywhere else.

Once the announcement of the tragic new cases had been released, the language began to shift. Gone were the blanket assurances, and in their place came statements that were slightly more equivocal. Significant qualifications began to creep into the dialogue. 'Scientists say there is no evidence of a link' became 'Scientists say that there is no *conclusive* evidence . . .' The persuasive blandishments about beef being 'perfectly safe' were subtly transmuted into 'safe, in the *normal sense* of the word'.

For journalists covering the story it was a frustrating experience. We have seen (Chapter 4) how one investigative reporter was told he was misguided and irresponsible when he was reporting the first cases in the series of cases the Government announced in March 1996. There are many other such examples. Many spokesmen have criticized the media. The impression was created that newspaper and television journalists were hell-bent on creating mischief and causing unwarranted anxiety amongst members of the public. In a television programme as this book goes to press, an Opposition spokesman shows how people have been convinced that scientists were not making warning noises. 'The public were always told beef was safe,' she said. 'It would have been more honest to admit that there simply wasn't any scientific opinion one way or the other.' So ingrained has this view become that even the Opposition believes it.

This view is false. From the first, scientists have been aware that there were possible risks. We said so in meetings, discussed it over a glass of wine, speculated on the possible consequences as events began to unfold. Why was the point not put in the public domain? It always was. The official reports, by scientists commissioned by the Government, raised a warning note time and time again. Their views were not passed on to the public.

The first major report was edited by Sir Richard Southwood, the Linacre Professor of Zoology at Oxford. Also on his committee was Professor Anthony Epstein, a distinguished virologist and Emeritus Professor of Pathology at Bristol. Dr Epstein was co-discoverer of the important Epstein-Barr virus, and an acknowledged authority on unusual virus diseases. There was Dr W. B. Martin, formerly Director of the Moredun Research Institute of Edinburgh and an eminent veterinarian, and Sir John Walton (now Lord Walton).

Was the Ministry hoping to obtain a gentle and non-critical document? There were some surprising absentees from the group they assembled. For example, there was no scrapie specialist from MAFF, and no world authority on kuru, CJD or prion diseases. One might also have hoped to see a member of the neuropathogenesis group at Edinburgh, where the CJD studies are centred.

Any thought that the selection of members might somehow dilute the conclusions was banished when the document was published. Here are some selected quotes from the original pages:

Southwood Report, February 1989*:

- Paragraph 5.3.1: 'With the very long incubation period of spongiform encephalopathies in humans, it may be a decade or more before complete reassurance can be given.'
- Paragraph 5.3.5: 'Because the possibility that BSE could be transmitted orally cannot be entirely ruled out, known affected cattle should not enter the human food chain . . .'
- Paragraph 5.3.6: 'It is a reasonable assumption that were BSE to be transmitted to humans, the clinical disorder would closely resemble CJD. Depending on the route of transmission, the incubation period could be as little as a year . . . or several decades [and] specialists . . . should be made aware of the emergence of BSE so that they can report any atypical cases or changing patterns in the incidence of disease.'
- Paragraph 9.2 (Conclusions): 'From the present evidence, it is most unlikely that BSE will have any implications for human health. Nevertheless, if our assessments of these likelihoods are incorrect, the implications would be extremely serious.'
- Paragraph 10.4 (Summary): 'Concerned at the remote chance that this new infection could be transmitted orally to man, we recommend the destruction of carcases of cattle with suspected BSE and prohibition of the use of milk from such cows for humans. These recommendations have already been acted upon.'

The bulk of this report was written during 1988, just one year after BSE was officially recognized. The Committee's judicious warnings were set out with perfect clarity. They said :

- They could give no reassurance for ten years or so;

*Southwood, Richard (editor), 1989, *Report of the Working Party on Bovine Spongiform Encephalopathy*, 35pp, London: Department of Health and Ministry of Agriculture, Fisheries & Food.

- They could not rule out the chance that BSE could be passed on in food;
- The disease could take over a decade to appear;
- Specialists should watch out for it.

It is obvious that they felt the present evidence was not conclusive, but they stated plainly firstly that they were 'concerned' at the possibility of transmission, and that if anything did happen the consequences would be 'extremely serious'. It is hard to imagine a more balanced and scientific appraisal.

No such open objectivity has ever been presented to the public by the government spokesmen. Let us move on six years, to a report chaired by David Tyrrell in 1994. Dr Tyrrell became known to the public through his research programme at the Common Cold Research Unit in Wiltshire, of which he was Director for many years. He emphasized that the 'results of all research should be open for scrutiny'. Here are some of the comments from his committee:

The Tyrrell Report of September 1994*:

- Page 9: We do not . . . comment on policy; that is not appropriate to the Committee.
- Page 36: Control measures are necessary for public health . . . because the BSE agent may be a human pathogen.
- Page 46: Human transmissible spongiform encephalopathy. As there were fears that meat products from BSE-infected cattle . . . might cause cases of CJD or a similar disease, it was decided to monitor human TSEs throughout the UK . . . It is too early to

* Tyrrell, David (editor) 1994, *Transmissible Spongiform Encephalopathies, a Summary of Present Knowledge and Research*, 99pp, London: HMSO.

> draw any conclusions because the incubation period in kuru, for example, can exceed 30 years.

These are comments made when the full extent of the BSE epidemic was clearly apparent. The most obvious difference between the tone of Dr Tyrrell's report and that of Sir David Southwood is the disclaimer in the opening pages: 'We do not comment on policy; that is not appropriate to the committee', we read in the preface. The words sound almost like official small print. There is no mistaking the warnings which the Committee expressed. In terms nobody could mistake, they emphasize:

- The BSE agent may cause human disease.
- Fears exist that BSE in cattle might cause something like CJD in people.
- Transmissible spongiform encephalopathy cases in Britain were to be monitored.
- Nine years after BSE was discovered it was still too early to draw conclusions.
- Human infections might take thirty years to appear.

Why were the public not told? These honest and perceptive sentiments were the conclusions of people who had immersed themselves in the subject. The Committee make it plain that they are drawing obvious conclusions based on the current state of understanding. I believe the public would have found the candour refreshing, for it reminds everyone that science is meant to be nothing more than a process of open assessment of the evidence available. I find the clarity of this report admirable, and regret that the public never knew.

Even when the subject is being examined in the abstract there are clear indications of the sense of concern felt by scientists in the field. One of the areas of investigation is into the role of prions, the minute fine threads which are found in the brain tissues of spongy-brain victims. The Royal Society of London held an important meeting on the subject in 1993. These specialists are concerned with the possible causes of these diseases, yet even in these detached lectures there are clear suggestions of the problems that might lie ahead.

Molecular Biology of Prion Diseases, published 1994*

- page 371: Considerable concern has been raised that the inclusion of BSE-infected meat and more specifically offal in the production of human foodstuffs may result in the transmission of BSE to humans, although there is no evidence for this at present.
- page 376: It remains to be seen if the dietary exposure to bovine prions will result in transmission to humans.

As the official spokesmen and politicians keep emphasizing, there is 'no scientific evidence' for any transmission of BSE to humans. Yet scientists do not confine themselves to commenting only on matters of certainty. The judicious speculation which has taken place ever since BSE was first identified shows that specialists, just like the public, have been thinking aloud about what might happen. Professor John Collinge heads the Prion Research Unit at Imperial College, London, and is in regular contact with research workers from many laboratories around the world. If the sense of their conclusions is extracted from this scientific paper there is no mistaking a feeling of foreboding:

*Collinge, John and Palmer, Mark S. (1994), Molecular genetics of human prion diseases, *Philosophical Transactions of the Royal Society of London* B 343: 371-378.

- Infected meat (especially offal) may result in BSE in people.
- The possibility has caused considerable concern.
- It remains to be seen if it happens.

Here I have presented comments from three publications. Between them, they cover the ground. There is an early committee report concerned with policy and the future of research, a recent report which isn't concerned with policy matters, and a specialized scientific meeting on molecular biology. The contributors range from experienced doctors to university professors. Some are dynamic and lively, others are quiet and reserved; some are well-known names, others are more obscure. They have all been wondering about the possible future of BSE, like everyone else in Britain, with the advantage that they are steeped in current research and regularly in contact with worldwide workers at the forefront of enquiry.

The comment that, as yet, we are short of firm scientific evidence for a causative link between BSE and human spongy-brain disease is clearly spelled out in each of these documents:

- 'From the evidence it is unlikely', said Southwood (1989)
- 'It remains to be seen', Collinge and Palmer concurred (1993)
- 'It is too early to draw conclusions', Tyrrell pointed out (1994)

We have heard about those comments, time and time again. Yet each document goes on to list the warning note that the Government should have sounded. Of those warnings, nothing more was heard. The Prime Minister has emphasized that the official confidence in the safety of beef stems from a lack of evidence for a link between infected beef and human spongy-brain disease, and likes to add that the facts are beyond dispute (Chapter 9). The lack of firm proof is, indeed, contested by no-one. But a sense of unease was widely published as well, yet nothing more was heard of it.

Television and the Cover-up

In 1992 a thriller serial was transmitted by BBC television. It concerned a farmer who catches BSE and told of a massive cover-up which surrounds this fictitious event. The *Radio Times* in May 1992 quoted the Government's chief veterinary officer, Mr Keith Meldrum. In response to critical comments arising from the programmes, Mr Meldrum said: 'It isn't possible for BSE to enter the human food chain.' A sense of doubt and a readiness to accept that there might be a link has regularly been conveyed by concerned scientists, and of that there is no sign in any of these official statements.

The money that goes into the scientific research is public money. We built the institutes, we pay the salaries. The resulting conclusions belong in the public domain, and were placed there by the scientists themselves. For official comments to select the good news, and only that, may be the way people play politics. But it is not the way we do science, and the Government must be made to realize that. Any suggestion that this growing body of knowledge might frighten the public is absurd. There have never been such blatant attempts to launder the truth when previous health warnings emerged. Young people know perfectly well that cigarettes might painfully kill them, but it has little effect on reducing the level of smoking. Business executives know that fatty foods threaten them with heart attacks, but you rarely see such people waving away a *filet mignon* and turning instead to salad. Young parents know that someone dies on the roads every hour or two, yet it has little effect on their setting out for a Sunday afternoon drive along the motorway. Nobody suggested that government propaganda should try to suppress those findings.

People take risks, they make judgements, and they are always interested to consider what the specialists think. In this area governmental thinking keeps public opinion and science at arm's length from each other. There can be no more timely reminder of the distance which separates the public from scientific reality.

If ever there was a case for bringing more scientists into the processes of government, this is it.

9

BEEF OFF THE MENU

Eloise is sixty. She was born and raised in Provence, but came to Cambridge in middle age and fell in love with England. Gracious and charming, she is alert to the realities of life in a modern world and has always followed health news with more than average interest. The French adore their food, and meat is a central ingredient of traditional French cooking. Like many visitors to England, Eloise was surprised at the quality of the best of British food. Roast beef and grilled steaks were a delight. Steak and kidney puddings became a continuing pleasure.

One aspect bothered her, and that was the trend towards high technology on the farm. The hormone treatment of cattle caused her concern, and she bought less beef in response to that. Reports of antibiotics in meat led to her reducing her purchases still further, and the continued use of intensive rearing of veal seemed unnecessarily inhumane. Then, in 1988, she read a small newspaper item about BSE. That was enough for Eloise. She fed the weekend's meat to the dog.

In April 1996 she heard about the first French patient believed to have died from the new spongy-brain disease, and that was the final straw. 'Now I will never taste wonderful English beef again,' she says with a regretful smile.

Beef Panic

The public response to the pronouncements on the young victims of the new human spongy-brain disease was predictable. Millions of families gave up beef overnight. Interest in vegetarianism exploded. Bookshops reported that their sales of vegetarian cookery books went up threefold within a couple of weeks. Sales of a book called *The Moosewood Cookbook*, something of a cult amongst connoisseurs of vegetarian cuisine, increased sixfold. Promotional displays about the joys of vegetarian cookery were everywhere and the springtime bookshops were as busy as they are at Christmas.

At the Vegetarian Society, membership enquiries doubled. At one stage in April 1996 they were sending out membership packs to enquirers at the rate of 200 per day. The effects of the scare were also felt at the Soil Association, which promotes organic agriculture. Their representatives said that the BSE scare had done more for their recruitment than all their promotional activities for the last decade. Currently, only 0.3 per cent of the usable land area of Britain is given over to organic farming, but that now seems set to increase. The demand for beef from organic farms, or from farmers who can be trusted to have fed nothing but vegetable matter to their herds, has been increasing by the day. Retail outlets for organic produce reported an increase of sales of 40 per cent in the week following the momentous announcement in the House of Commons.

Official action against BSE-infected beef is not new. Some individuals have felt inclined to avoid British beef throughout the saga of BSE, and official policies have often followed in the wake of personal pronouncements. Suggestions that nerve tissues might be banned from human consumption had been circulating ever since the BSE agent had been located in the central nervous system of cattle.

The regulations were slow to change, until June 1989 when Dr Hugh Fraser of the Institute of Animal Health announced that he and several colleagues would no longer be eating any sausages, pies, or other foods that might contain such ingredients. The Ministry was obliged to consider this seriously, and after a five-month consultation period they did agree to impose a ban on the use of these foods in products for human consumption. Dr Fraser, meanwhile, was officially told to keep his views to himself in future.

Beef is Banned in School

Public concern soon focused on school meals. The prospect of young people being exposed to an infective agent about which little was known came to predominate in discussions in education departments across the country. Many decided to play safe. The first authority to ban British beef from the school menu was Humberside county council. After considering the reports, they decided to take this step in 1990. Roast beef and other beef meals had been a tradition at schools in the area. In Yorkshire villages with names like Pocklington Wolgate traditional British beef is just what you would expect. But the pupils in the local school, along with the other 470 schools under the authority, sat down to their first lunch in an era without British beef products on 14 May 1990.

The beef in their spaghetti meals and mince for their

lasagne came instead from Africa. As local farmers bemoaned the lack of sales in this lucrative market, cattle raised by tribesmen in Botswana were supplying the Humberside schools with the beef for their school dinners. Shropshire schools soon followed, and within a few years the number of schools banning British beef products was in the thousands.

The supermarkets were quick to respond by erecting signs to reassure the public. In May 1990, after the adverse publicity, Safeway issued a categorical denial that any of their suppliers had a case of BSE. Sainsburys gave an absolute guarantee as well. When it was pointed out that, since there was no test, some animals free of symptoms might already have the infection, these were withdrawn. St Michael meat and sausages were said, by Marks & Spencer, to be free from 'any part of the animal implicated in the BSE mad cow disease' *(sic)*. They explained to reporters that this was because the implicated parts didn't include red meat, which is what they were selling.

Harrods came out with a judiciously worded reassurance which read: 'Harrods wishes to confirm that meat purchased for sale on these premises has been certified free from the symptoms of BSE', which set out matters as diplomatically as they could. During the early 1990s the sense of concern increased. Several dairy farmers had gone down with CJD. This turned out to be coincidence, but then there came reports of two teenagers ill with a form of the disease.

'Eat and Survive!'

Matters came to a head late in 1995 when the Prime Minister launched an 'eat and survive' campaign. On the afternoon of 6 December in the House of Commons,

John Major said this: 'There is currently no scientific evidence that BSE can be transmitted to humans, or that eating beef causes CJD in humans. That issue is not in question. I am also advised that beef is a safe and wholesome product.'

These reassurances had little effect on restoring public confidence. John Davis, of the Local Authority Caterers Association, launched a recommendation that all local authorities look again at beef fed to the youngsters in their care. They did not seek to proscribe all beef. He said, 'Our concern is in relation to some products made with mechanically recovered meat, MRM, which is meat taken off the bones by machine. Many authorities imposed this ban years ago, and we are now advising everyone to do it.'

As he was speaking the authorities were discussing a ban on mechanically recovered meat from bones associated with the central nervous system (the ban came into effect over Christmas 1995) but questions still persisted about the wisdom of permitting calves' brains into the human food supply. The justification for doing so was that the calves were too young to have acquired the agent of BSE from eating contaminated meal. There remained a chance that they might have acquired the disease direct from their mothers (through the placenta, or through milk). For this reason there were critics who pressed for calves' brains to be included in the ban. But calves' brains continued to be used.

The assurances given by the authorities do not always match reality. Dr John Pattison, adviser to the Government on BSE, is among those who have emphasized that the suspected organs of cows with BSE have been banned from the human food supply since 1989. Officially, that is the case. What is less often admitted is that the ban followed unilateral action by specialists like Dr Fraser to exclude pies and sausages from their own diets.

Not much is said about the failure of the ban to work in practice. Although the exclusion of brain and spinal cord was introduced in 1989, there were so many reports that the rules were not being followed that they were tightened up in November 1995. A further review of the controls took place in April 1996. The need for the regulations to receive this kind of periodic adjustment did not confirm, in the minds of the public, that the Government had known what it was doing in the first place.

The newspaper headlines confirmed the sense of unease. 'Beef prices plummet in BSE scare' said one; 'Schools in rush to outlaw beef', said another. One plaintive call echoed a question in many minds: 'Beef: who can we believe?' There had been numerous attempts to assuage public anxiety. The best-known, and certainly the most counter-productive, was a published photograph of John Selwyn Gummer (the then Minister of Agriculture) giving his daughter Cordelia a hamburger to bite. In the words of the press she was 'force-fed' the burger by her father, and the television film of the event seems to confirm this. I may be wrong, but the impression I formed after watching it a couple of times was that the young girl did not really want it, and she does not appear actually to eat any. If that's the case, she was wiser by far than her father.

Mr Gummer was reminded of his folly of six years earlier in a radio interview during April 1996. Did he regret the incident, in the light of the recent cases? He was incandescent with anger. How dare the BBC pose such a question. If they wished to know about agricultural matters they should ask the current Minister, and not him. His answer was so uncompromising and so firm that I felt a certain sense of admiration. The interviewer, James Naughtie, could well have responded by a teasing remark about the personal nature of the event, and the individual purpose of the question; but he missed the chance and was lost for words. It was one up to the Minister. I only hope Cordelia feels the same.

The crucial turning-point in the subject came with the ban of meat and bone-meal from animal feeds. From that moment on the number of new cases in calves born after the ban (and known as BABs) declined steadily.

25,690	cases born after feed ban, July 1988
11,129	born in last half of 1988
10,413	born in 1989
3,140	born in 1990
957	born in 1991
50	born in 1992
1	born in 1993

Table 9: Animals with BSE Born after the Ban (BABs)

After the Government's announcement on 20 March 1996 many people felt it was an end for the beef industry in Britain. Over 700 workers were immediately laid off in Northern Ireland alone. Demand for beef fell by 90 per cent that day. It has not recovered; even at their best, sales have remained 15 per cent below the normal level.

Hamburgers for Ever

The adverse reports about beef did not affect everyone, however. A journalist from *The Times* went out to report on the way children were reacting. She found that if you offered youngsters a choice of hamburgers or chicken pie, nine out of ten still went for the burger. A seven-year-old pointedly asked the headteacher at a Hampshire school what the fuss was about, and had a reasoned reply about the new doubts over the safety of British beef.

The news had no effect whatever on the children, who carried on munching their burgers unconcerned. When pressed, the headteacher said he had received just one phone call from an anxious parent about beef on the menu. This was two days after the Government's statement about the new cases of spongy-brain disease in young adults. He explained that beef remained on the menu at Hampshire schools, always with an alternative. And he added, 'I always eat beef myself.'

For the parents it proved to be a difficult matter. The concept of mealtime as a leisurely and relaxed family event is gone, for most youngsters. For them, the American idea of fast food predominates, and a meal has become more of a pit-stop for refuelling. Why are hamburgers so popular? They have become the favourite American quick meal during the twentieth century, and reflect ancient European traditions. Hamburgers are named from the German town of Hamburg. They have nothing to do with ham (the popular term 'beefburger' is a response which may assist sales to sectors of society who don't eat pig meat).

There are many German recipes for chopped steaks, sometimes blended with a little egg, onion or herbs. They are popularly known as *Hacksteaks*. Without doubt the best way to make a hamburger is to chop good steak at home, blend in a little beaten egg and chopped onion, pat it into shape with washed hands, and then cook it at high heat on a bake-stone or thick iron pan with little fat. The product is like a braised steak, except that the chopping process allows the cook to use cheaper cuts than would otherwise be the case. The hamburger roll is an American version of the European tradition of eating such meats with bread.

Once the product is in the roll, you can't see what went inside. Manufacturers know that, and with the continuing popularity of burger products they are always keen to cut costs if they can. The cheapest such products are made with cereal binder and mechanically recovered meat. The extent of these forms of beef in modern foods is hard to imagine, but a freezer at home may contain pizzas and pies, lasagne and minced meat, sausages and hamburger steaks. In everything but the pizza there is likely to be beef, and in budget-priced items the likelihood of recovered meat and other bulking ingredients is that much higher.

The value of beef sales in British supermarkets adds up to £1.8 million per year. Beef is big business. The trend towards exploiting mechanically recovered meat (MRM) was led by the mass consumers of beef products, like the supermarkets and the burger chains, who were determined to minimize their costs. The rival burger chains, including McDonald's, Burger King and Wimpy, said that the official announcements about the risks from beef had negligible effect on sales. None the less, a major chain announced a cessation of burger production whilst they consolidated their supplies exclusively from non-British sources. Was this done for scientific reasons? No, said their chief executive, it was done because of customer demand. There were few signs of disillusioned customers, it must be said; preserving market share and claiming some headline attention might also have been motives behind the move. It is only because of the great purchasing conglomerates that the pressure to exploit products like MRM existed in the first place.

The decision to use imported beef caused new problems. Black-market drugs, fattening agents, hormones and antibiotics are still illegally used in some areas of Western Europe. The Latin nations in particular are less likely to conform to every official rule and regulation, and the culture of these lands is very different from that of Britain where animal welfare is concerned. One young vet tells me he visited slaughterhouses around the

Mediterranean to obtain an indication of how animal slaughter was handled in the different countries. 'Some of the things I saw were horrible,' he said. 'There's hardly anyone to whom I would show the video. The things they do to animals would turn your stomach.'

The amount of illegally-reared beef that has been imported in Britain since late March 1996 has considerably increased. The meat now provided by the organizations which imposed a ban on British beef brings in its wake poor standards of rearing, lowered standards of safety, and almost non-existent levels of humane treatment for the cattle. There is an added problem. Britain has exported many thousands of cattle to Europe over the years. There is every chance that the hamburger giants are re-importing British beef from the Continent.

10

THE WORLD REACTS

The announcement that ten young people had died with an unrecognized form of spongy-brain disease erupted in the House of Commons on the afternoon of 20 March 1996 with all the effect of an abdication, an assassination or a terrorist attack. None of the cautious warnings from the committee reports had been quoted by spokesmen in the past. The continuing reassurance that there were no problems had lulled Parliament into a sense of smug security about beef. Now that these assurances had been dashed, panic set in.

The meat industry closed down overnight. Slaughterhouses stayed shut until the beginning of April. The suddenness of the announcement and the sense of 'about face' was bewildering. On one hand lay unease within the ranks of farmers, vets and the retail trade, for one of our largest industries was facing calamity. It seemed necessary to keep hold on reality, because everywhere there was a sense of public anxiety, and little information was ready to pass to the public. Announcements were confused.

Farmers, faced with animals who were ready for

slaughter, could not send them to market. In one West Country sale healthy calves were sold at £1 for three. Cattle are produced on a continuous timetable, and keeping those destined for slaughter posed further problems. They all needed feeding and the late spring meant there was insufficient grass to feed them out of doors.

At Last: an Admission

The Health Secretary Stephen Dorrell told the House of Commons that the most likely explanation for the ten cases was now believed to be exposure to BSE before the specified offal ban had been introduced in 1989. Two points should be made about this. First (and the Minister reminded the Commons of the fact) there was no scientific evidence for the link. Having denied for years that there was any risk at all, it was almost as though the Government's advisers were forced into conceding a connection without much evidence to back it up.

The second aspect was the effectiveness of the ban. As we have seen, the regulations have not worked. Half the slaughterhouses in Britain did not carry out the controls properly. Contaminated offal was still getting into the food supply years after the ban was introduced. The nature of the risk was pure guesswork; but meanwhile the existence of the regulations was used to cover up the reality.

Two additional safety precautions were announced by the Government. On the afternoon of 20 March Mr Douglas Hogg, the Minister for Agriculture, told the House of Commons that meat and bone-meal, which were still being used in agriculture, would be banned and that there would be further attempts to separate meat from waste in older cattle. His announcement introduced these new measures:

- Meat from animals aged over thirty months must be deboned before sale.
- All meat and bone-meal will be banned for sale as pig and poultry feed.

Concerns about the safety of meal in animal feed were ended, for the use of all such meal was finished. It was ten years since the disease was first recognized, and at last the suspect feed had been banned.

The effects on the British economy looked as though they would be severe. The meat industry supports 41,000 dairy farmers and 95,000 farmers raising beef. In total it is worth £4 billion a year. Half of all farmers earn all or part of their income from cattle. Last year Britain exported 242,000 tonnes of beef worth £520 million. Mr Dorrell added: 'There are major and legitimate economic interests, jobs, associated with the industry, but the paramount responsibility must be the protection of human health.' There was a hollow sound in those words to everyone who knew how poorly the offal ban had been implemented, and how funds were being kept back from research into BSE and from the implementation of MAFF's own safety controls.

The French move against Britain

First to move against British beef was France. The French have long been the largest importer, with over 90,000 tonnes a year being sent across the Channel. The trade is worth £220 million per year. All cattle from British stock were quarantined, and the herds where the sixteen admitted French outbreaks had occurred – mostly in Brittany – were slaughtered. Belgium, Holland, Portugal and Sweden quickly followed with bans of their own. A German spokesman announced: 'In the light of the new information, the aim must be to secure a general export ban on British meat, meat products, offal, animal meal and raw materials for pharmaceuticals and cosmetics in the European Union.' The British authorities complained that the bans were illegal, and Brussels began making sympathetic public noises in support. Privately, the European Union were already planning to make the ban official within a week.

As luck would have it, the next day had been chosen for a promotional lunch for Scottish beef in Paris. The event had been sponsored by 'Food From Britain' in conjunction with an association of fifty top restaurants across France. It took place in Bertie's, a celebrated British restaurant which had even brought in a kilted bagpiper for the occasion. The sole topic of conversation was the newly reported risks of eating British beef.

In Britain, matters moved so fast that statements of reassurance kept contradicting themselves. The National Farmers Union issued a statement on 25 March which said:

> 'The NFU welcome the decision of SEAC (the Spongiform Encephalopathy Advisory Group) that no additional measures are necessary at this stage to protect public health.'

Even as this was being released, pressure was building up for action over meat from older dairy cattle, and on 26 March (the very next day) the NFU published a new statement with a very different tone:

> 'The NFU is demanding the introduction of a special scheme to take older cows out of the food chain to restore consumer confidence in British beef.'

This was a foolish reversal of opinion, and seems to have been issued to keep in favour with the way government thinking was already beginning to move. Farmers (no matter what their union might be saying) were most unwilling to opt for the slaughter of all cows of a certain age, even if perfectly healthy.

Once the fears had been officially broadcast, international intervention was soon on the scene. Britain tried to insist that there were no serious worries and trade should continue as before, with the new safeguards in action. One British member of the European Parliament waved a bag of jelly babies to illustrate the implications of a complete ban on all beef products. But the Austrian Agricultural Commissioner Franz Fischler stated that there was now a crisis of confidence in British beef which had to be addressed.

Europe's Official Ban

The European Commission imposed a world ban on British beef on 27 March 1996. Many British voices questioned whether a ban outside the EU could be lawful, but the Commission emphasized that this was necessary or dealers would simply export to non-EU nations and then re-import as though nothing had happened. A world trading ban was the only answer. These were their requirements:

- As an emergency measure, the transport of all cattle and all beef products from the United Kingdom to the other member states would be banned, and these provisions shall also apply to export to non-member countries to prevent deflections of trade.
- The Commission will carry out in the coming weeks a Community inspection across the United Kingdom to evaluate the application of the measures taken.
- The significance of new information and the measures taken must be subjected to detailed scientific study.

- The decision will be reviewed once all the above elements have been examined.

As expected, the European Union stepped in officially to ban all British beef and beef products. This included gelatine and the full list of meat products (Chapter 6). The export of some popular chocolate products, biscuits and sweets was immediately halted. Because of the widespread use of beef products (such as gelatine) the banned goods included such stalwarts as Curly Wurlies, Mini Eggs and Strollers. British yoghurt was banned, along with lipstick and soap, ice-cream and medicinal capsules. The official categories of banned exports were these:

- All meat of bovine animals slaughtered in the United Kingdom;
- Products obtained from these animals which may enter the animal or human food chain and materials destined for use in medicinal, cosmetic or pharmaceutical products;
- Mammalian-derived meat and bone-meal;
- Live bovine animals, their semen and embryos.

The British government issued a statement in which an emergency package was set out. It was intended to cushion the industry from the imposition of controls by Brussels. The sudden panic over the safety of beef had meant that slaughterhouses became inactive overnight, and closures were imminent without aid.

- £1.5 million per week was allocated to the rendering industry which disposes of slaughterhouse wastes. This subsidy will help preserve 3,000 jobs. This assistance is described as 'temporary but vital short-term aid'.
- £50 million was made available for the slaughter of young bull calves produced from dairy cows. These are the veal calves affected by the export ban, and if fattened would add to the beef surplus.

- A further £15 million is to be paid to livestock farmers. The premium payments made to farmers would total £170 million (compared with £135 million in 1995).

The banning of British beef from world trade had far-reaching implications. Because of its quality and reliability, it has long been in demand and some breeds (like the Aberdeen Angus) are known even in the Far East. The latest export figures give a clear indication of the importance of the business:

Nation	Annual total of British beef (tonnes)
France	98,000
Italy	27,200
South Africa	27,100
Ireland	24,100
Netherlands	17,800
Spain	5,600
Denmark	4,600
Benelux	3,850
Portugal	2,900
Mauritius	2,500
Ghana	2,300
Angola	1,800
Malta	1,700
Saudi Arabia	1,700
Germany	1,600
Hungary	1,600
Philippines	1,500
Sweden	1,500
Hong Kong	1,300
Greece	250
Austria	4

Table 10: World Markets for British Beef

By the end of March 1996 the total cost of the mad cow crisis to Brussels stood at £2.5 billion. Britain's reputation abroad was hit hard. The former European Commission President Jacques Delors said that the affair was caused entirely by muddled governmental action in Britain. 'One Minister said everything was all right, while another said the situation was very dangerous,' he remarked.

To settle the extent of European commitments, the European Commissioner Sir Leon Brittan agreed to appear on the *Breakfast with Frost* programme on BBC television. Could he clarify exactly how much support British agriculture could expect from Brussels? 'Different schemes get different cooperation,' he said, 'which ranges from 100 per cent, to 70 per cent, to 50 per cent.'

On 31 March Douglas Hogg went to Europe with a proposal for the slaughter and incineration of cattle on an unprecedented scale. He asked for 80 per cent of the cost to be borne by the European Union. The French Agriculture Minister Phillippe Vasseur said he regarded this as merely the opening bid in a round of negotiations. Johen Borchert from Germany said that he thought 70 per cent was more like it. He referred to a recent outbreak of swine fever in Germany, where European money had also been sought to help compensate farmers. At that time, Britain had insisted that financial support to Germany should be kept as low as possible. The 70 per cent share is what Germany had been allowed during their own crisis. Another British commissioner, Neil Kinnock, warned that, whatever was offered, half the payments would be clawed back next year anyway.

The episode was harmful to British relationships right across Europe. Television coverage was critical of official responses, most notably of the Government's failure to adopt a coordinated and scientific stance. Newspapers from around Europe showed how reporters viewed the situation when the export ban was imposed:

- **Austria:** 'This is part of the unstoppable decline of the Tory Prime Minister John Major,' said the *Kurier.*
- **Belgium:** 'Mad cows contaminate the political climate of Europe,' reported *Le Soir.*
- **France:** 'Mr Major and his government have not even managed to persuade their own citizens,' *Le Parisien.*
- **Germany:** 'It was surprising to see the coldness and toughness with which the British are playing their game of "one against all",' *Frankfurter Allgemeine.*
- **Holland:** 'Relations between Britain and the rest of Europe have sunk to a historically low level,' *De Telegraaf.*
- **Italy:** 'Panic stormed Downing Street after British technologists failed to convince the European Union,' concluded *La Repubblica.*
- **Spain:** 'The British delegation to the EU have not done their homework. The decision to keep the embargo on British cows fell like a jug of cold water on the hopes of the British government,' *El Pais.*
- **Norway:** 'The uproar over BSE in Britain clearly has more to do with trust and political honesty than with food or drugs,' concluded *Aftenposten.*

There was one fundamental question in all this, which nobody had raised. If British beef posed such a problem to health, why were the British still allowed to eat it? If it was not good enough for mainland Europe, should it not be banned from domestic sale as well? Though no-one said so, the ban was introduced simply to allow the rest of Europe to keep exporting. No European official believed that British beef was dangerous. As I have said, it is certain that suspect beef is already in Europe, and is being exported under other guises.

The political importance of a ban did not become

clear until 15 April, when the newspapers reported comments by the Agriculture Commissioner Franz Fischler. Had he believed British beef was a hazard? 'No,' he said. 'If we thought that, its sale would have to be banned in Britain as well as elsewhere.' So, what did he feel personally about medical risks? 'I would not hesitate to eat beef in England,' he replied. 'I know no medical reason not to.'

The Market Collapse

In the British shops, meanwhile, no-one yet knew of the private views that were driving Brussels. Prices of beef plummeted. Minced meat, normally on sale for £1.50 a pound, fell to one-tenth of the price. Even at 15p a pound, which it reached on 25 March, there were few takers. One butcher, who expected to take £600 from sales of beef in a day, sold scraps of meat and mince worth no more than £50. Like many other butchers, he sold not a single piece of roasting beef for the weekend of 23 March. Lamb, chicken and pork, meanwhile, sold in record amounts. Many markets were closed. Hereford market on the following Monday had not a single buyer or seller turn up. One of the biggest markets of all, at Hexham in Northumberland, stayed closed as the week commenced.

The episode ended almost as soon as it started, for the supermarkets stepped in to maintain cash flow. It's interesting to note that they did not discard what many people by now regarded as 'contaminated' supplies, but instead they slashed prices in order to keep selling. After a week of worry, the public were willing to capitalize on the retailers' response. There was a record boom in sales as shoppers bought up half-price beef and put it away in freezer cabinets at home. Saturday 30 March was the first day when Sainsburys sold out of beef in all their 363 stores.

At the month's end, average sales of beef had been just a little lower than would have been expected. Roast beef remained on the menu. Beef farmers, who know more than most, were eating their beef and wondering why their world seemed about to end. In the Midlands, meanwhile, the news about beef gave a bonus to a little-known British food industry, the sale of horse-meat. One horse butcher in Smethwick sells horse-meat at 20p–80p per pound. Until recently he charged £70 to collect and dispose of a horse carcase.

Now (if a vet will issue a certificate that the animal is fit for human consumption) he will collect them free. Or at a discount, at least.

11

WHAT ARE THE RISKS FROM BSE?

It was hot in the television studio, nearing the end of a long day. The interview was live. There was one final point I wished to prove – how strong were our controls on germs in people, but how lax they were when the germs were the subject of scientific study. As the item neared its end I put my hand in my pocket and brought out a bottle of typhoid. I set the culture of the bacilli on the table in front of a startled Ludovic Kennedy. Never have I seen him quite so surprised.

There were then no controls on the handling of dangerous germs. Ever since the dawn of microbiology three hundred years ago, research was done without any formal regulation of the way germs were handled. As a youngster I had a year working with dangerous bacteria as a junior member of staff of the Medical Research Council, and was amazed at the lack of controls on the way bacteria were studied, and the possible hazards to staff. By the 1970s the matter was becoming increasingly urgent, and I published a proposal that organisms should be categorized according to the risk they posed to people. The response in the studio to that culture bottle of typhoid, growing on egg medium, was a timely reminder of the hazards we faced. If the same bacteria had been living in my gall-bladder, rather than in my pocket, I could have been detained on the spot. There were no controls at all on what you did with a culture. As an easy subject for the attention of terrorists, pathogenic microbes were strangely neglected.

The first paper setting out my proposals for legal safeguards was called 'No legal control of biological hazards', and was published in the *New Law Journal*. It was followed by a number of newspaper reports, including an editorial in *The Times* of London, and I subsequently outlined the proposal at greater length in a leading article, 'Call for Biohazard Legislation', for the scientific journal *Nature*.

Papers and Reports on the Control of how Germs are Handled

Ford, Brian J., 1971, No Legal Control of Biological Hazards, PUBLIC HEALTH, *New Law Journal,* **121** (5511): 823-824, 16 September.

Report, 1971, Disease 'risk' in Labs, *Guardian*, 17 September.

Berlins, Marcel, and Wright, Pearce, 1971, Call for Law to Control Laboratory Poisons, *The Times*, 17 September.

Report, 1973, Absence of regulations for Microbes is risk to Public Health, expert says, *The Times,* 11 April.

Anon, 1973, The Case for a Far Wider Enquiry [leader in support of campaign], *The Times,* 18 April.

Report, 1973, Author repeats Microbe warning, *South Wales Echo,* 11 April.

Ford, Brian J., 1973, *The Proposal for Biohazard Legislation: Its Implications for Microscopy,* Inter-Micro 73, King's College, Cambridge, 20 July.

——, 1973, 'Regrettable Episodes of infection ...' [in] *Optical Microscope Manual*: 196, London: Harrap, Sydney and Auckland: Reed International.

——, 1973, Biohazard Law, [in] *The Revealing Lens: Mankind and the Microscope*: 201-202, London: Harrap, September.

——, 1974, Call for Biohazard Legislation, *Nature,* **250**: 364-365, 2 August.

Glick, J. L., 1976, Reflections and Speculations on Regulation of Molecular Genetic Research [quotes 'BIOHAZARD' paper, 2 August 1974, *Nature*], *Annals of the New York Academy of Science:* 178 et seq., June.

From this came official legislation, and the concept has since been embodied in codes of conduct around the world. The culturing of germs and the handling of the cultures is controlled, and episodes of disease contracted by scientists are kept to a minimum. The concept has backfired on occasions, I have to say; more than once I have been reminded to button up my white coat in a laboratory, and it would be easy to feel tempted to resent such regulations, until I stop to think that this was originally my proposal in the first place.

Spongy-brain disease agents pose new problems, and a special report was commissioned by the Advisory

Committee on Dangerous Pathogens to set out safe procedures for research on BSE and the related infections. The spongy-brain agents present us with special difficulties because of the high temperatures necessary to inactivate them, and also because of this peculiar ability to resist disinfectants. The spongy-brain diseases that are genetically determined, and which we believe cannot be spread by infection, are excluded from this list. Infectivity was the criterion for inclusion.

Human:	Creutzfeldt-Jakob disease Gerstmann-Sträußler-Scheinker syndrome Kuru
Animal:	Scrapie – in sheep, goats and moufflon Bovine spongiform encephalopathy Transmissible mink encephalopathy Chronic wasting disease in deer and elk Feline spongiform encephalopathy (cats, cheetahs, etc.) Spongiform encephalopathy in zoo antelopes (kudu, oryx, etc.)

Table 11: Transmissible spongy-brain diseases

The existence of these infective agents is well-known, and in the case of scrapie has been mentioned for centuries. What remains puzzling is the extraordinarily resistant nature of the infective principle, whatever it is. Cooking does not destroy it, as we have already seen, nor do conventional disinfectants. Every known germ is killed in an autoclave, a laboratory-scale pressure-cooker, if exposed to temperatures of 121°C for fifteen minutes. That is always worth remembering, for a pressure-cooker at home is the perfect way to sterilize heat-resistant materials if someone has been ill with food poisoning. Spongy-brain agents are unaffected by this treatment.

They resist even nuclear radiation. Samples have been treated with ultraviolet radiation, and also exposed to gamma rays. These experiments show that the infectivity can come through unscathed.

It even survives in soil, for samples have been found to be infective years after burial. This has caused some anxiety over carcases which have been buried, using the JCB digger normally used for laying drains and digging ditches, rather than burned. What happens to the remains of cattle buried in this way? The question of the safety of water supplies needs to be considered. Organic material can always leach into water-courses, and some scare stories have circulated which suggest that there may be a future risk from tap water.

There is a grave of 100 headless cattle carcases buried in a land-fill site half a mile from the River Wensum from which the East Anglian city of Norwich draws its water. The supply company, Anglian Water, and the Environmental Agency are satisfied that the water supply cannot be infected. Their confidence stems from the fact that they have boreholes which are checked at least once a month, and so far no leaching from the site has been detected.

The practice of illicit burial is said to be more widespread in France. One French farmer said, knowingly, 'BSE, in French, means JCB.'

Some cases of CJD have been spread by doctors. In Britain there have been about twenty in all, extending over a quarter of a century. These people caught spongy-brain disease through hormone treatment or surgery.

Human Growth Hormone (hGH)

The first treatments with human growth hormone, hGH, were used to help those whose pituitary glands didn't function properly. These patients had developed slowly, and needed urgent intervention if they were ever to reach normal size. The hormone was taken from pituitary glands removed at post-mortem operations. Nobody suspected it at the time, but it now seems that some of the corpses from which the glands had been taken must have been carriers of CJD. A total of 1,981 people were treated with this hormone preparation, the last being in 1985. Ten British patients treated with the hGH died of CJD.

Human gonadotrophin (hPG)

This hormone was also extracted from pituitary glands. It was used to treat women during the 1970s. Four Australian women later died of CJD, believed to have been contracted from these injections. No cases occurred in Britain.

Corneal grafts

The transplant of a clear cornea into an eye damaged by disease is one way of restoring sight to the blind. The eye originally develops from nervous tissues in the embryo, and we believe that the agent of CJD can exist in the eye. In one case a patient developed CJD after a corneal transplant in 1974. No further cases have been recorded.

Brain membranes

A few cases have been recorded in which patients have picked up the infection from grafts of *dura mater*, the tissue covering the brain. This has been done when brain damage needed repair. The incubation period following the operation ranged from two to ten years.

Brain surgery

During the 1950s several patients developed CJD after brain surgery. We now believe that the instruments were still contaminated after use on a CJD patient. All the normal sterilization procedures were properly followed, but the agent survived. The levels of heat that sterilize instruments do not affect the infective principle of the spongy-brain diseases, nor do conventional disinfectants.

Laboratory infections

There are no records of this having happened. A few cases are known where laboratory workers died of CJD, and one pathologist is on record of being killed by this disease. There is no reason to suppose the infection was picked up in the laboratory, and the rate of incidence of the disease in pathologists and laboratory technicians is still said to be no higher, on average, than in the rest of the population.

The potential extent of the threat, and the first indication that the world of finance was taking it seriously, came within a week of the momentous announcement to the House of Commons. Before March was out the first insurance policy for BSE was announced. It was developed at the London brokers Goodfellow Rebecca Ingrams Pearson (GRIP). The proposal is for an annual premium of £10 per adult, or £20 for a family of four. The benefits are £25,000 for the adults and £2,500 in respect of children, payable on diagnosis of Creutzfeldt-Jakob disease, CJD. The premiums can be multiplied up to ten times, so the maximum pay-out on diagnosis could be £250,000. The company excluded issuing the policy to people working at a slaughterhouse or knackers' yard, but there was no exclusion on account of eating beef in the diet. People who work on meat counters in supermarkets, or serving hamburgers in a fast-food outlet, are all eligible.

The insurers were inundated with requests. A large newspaper company asked for details, describing the idea as 'brilliant'. A major international hamburger seller made contact, asking for full details. Over 40,000 policies were immediately ordered by a building society for their workforce.

How Great are the Dangers?

The danger of the agent lies in its relative indestructibility. Few normal processes will inactivate it. Against that we have to set the difficulty of catching it through contagion. These agents are not spread by contact, as far as we know. The risk from contaminated tissues varies from type to type. Brain and central nervous tissues are known to harbour the agent, whereas none has ever been found in beef. It has proved to be easy and repeatable to pass spongy-brain disease to rats and mice using nerve tissues, but attempts to pass an infection from meat from cows, like steak have not been successful. The report on the safe handling of the spongiform encephalopathy sets down the tissues in order of their possible risk:

a: Specified offals under the BSE Order 1991

Brain	Spinal cord	Spleen
Thymus	Tonsil	Lymph glands around the gut

b: Tissues that have been shown to contain high levels of infection

Pituitary gland	*Dura mater*	Placenta and membranes
Eye	Peripheral lymph nodes	

c: Tissues with small risk of infection

Major peripheral nerves	Pancreas
Adrenal glands	Lung

Cerebro-spinal fluid (CSF, from around the brain and spinal cord)

Liver

d: Believed very unlikely to carry infection

Milk	Saliva	Skin
Semen	Urine	Muscle
Faeces	Kidney	Blood*

**There is believed to be negligible risk from blood transfusion. Lymph cells accidentally injected could pose a significant hazard.*

Table 12: Distribution of Spongiform Encephalopathy agent in tissues

Because of the affinity of the agent for nerve tissue (bearing in mind that the eye develops from the nervous tissues of the embryo) the splashing of agent onto the eye may present a hazard. Since 1992, the dissection of eyes from cattle has been banned in British schools.

The requirements now recommended for the handling of specimens are these:

Basic safety precautions

- Protect skin wounds and eczema by using dressings
- Wear disposable gowns and gloves
- Wear eye-protectors
- Use enclosed systems when mixing or liquidizing specimens
- Never use sharp objects (needles, scalpels) unless necessary, handle them carefully
- Dispose of waste safely using double bags and incineration
- Re-use durable items only after special sterilization
- Decontaminate surfaces thoroughly
- Record all accidents, spillages, contamination, etc.

All such work is now supposed to be done in cabinets within laboratories dedicated for this type of research. Sterilizing equipment is not easy. The normal pressure-cooking (autoclave) temperatures don't work. A temperature of 132°C for an hour has been said to sterilize infected material in an autoclave, though some reports suggest even this is not always enough. Dry heat of 240°C for a minute or two greatly reduces the infectivity, but even this does not get rid of it altogether. A temperature of 200°C for an hour will inactivate the infectivity of moist tissues, but freeze-dried specimens can remain infectious even after an hour at 360°C. Routine disinfectants don't work, either.

Alcohols	Ethylene oxide
Formalin	Formaldehyde
Glutaraldehyde	Hydrogen peroxide
Iodophors	Phenolics
β-propiolactone	

Table 13: Disinfectants that are ineffective against spongy-brain infection

The only reliable disinfectant is bleach. Hypochlorite bleaches, if they can be strong enough to provide 20,000 parts per million of chlorine – which is very strong – can inactivate the agent. This is what must be used for bench surfaces. The only safe method of disposal for contaminated objects is incineration.

Spongy-brain agents are unlike any other form of germ. None of our normal methods of disinfection will work. I shall breathe a great sigh of relief when the incidence has been firmly controlled, and scrapie, like the other diseases, is no more.

Parsimony perpetuates Problems

One of the greatest problems that has been encountered stems from the Treasury. There is a lack of positive thinking which could have helped bring in suspect cows, and contaminated feed, far earlier. One recent legislative control was the ban of contaminated feed, which has been used up to 1996 for pigs, chickens and on fish farms. One objection to that is that the ban came too late. Far more to the point is that the Treasury has offered no financial compensation for those who have stocks of the feed, or of the meal from which it is made. There must be tens of thousands of tonnes of this contaminated feed in stores around Britain. What are people supposed to do? They have bought it, and paid the price, and have now been told to buy more for their animals. Meanwhile the contaminated meal lies around with nowhere to go. Even if it were to be written off by the owner and dumped, it would go straight into nature's food chain. What we need to do is to compensate people for bringing it in for incineration. The Treasury have got to understand that, if the Government wants people to help it clean up its own difficulties, it cannot be at the individual's cost. We have paid enough already.

We could have known more about these agents, and sooner, if more research had been properly funded when the epidemic was gaining ground. A proposal for a major programme of investigation was made in 1991 by Dr Stan Prusiner, Professor of Neurology at the University of California, San Francisco. Professor Prusiner is the scientist who coined the term 'prion' in 1982. He planned to cooperate with Dr Gareth Roberts, then at St Mary's Hospital, Paddington, in an investigation of the potential danger to the public of BSE. Professor Prusiner is the pioneer of the prion hypothesis, currently the favoured theory of the cause of spongy-brain diseases (Chapter 14). The modest proposal was refused. Ironically, the major meeting on the molecular biology of these diseases was held in London late in 1993. Professor Prusiner was an author of *four* of the papers presented at the meeting. His research has long been at the forefront in the field. The programme of research he had in mind is now starting at Imperial College, London. The delay has set back progress by years.

The fact that we lost out on a rare source of insight, at such a crucial time, shows how radically we need to change the relationship between science and government. The cost of the research programme would have been £3 million, at a time when the total budget for BSE research was £9 million. Within the last year, a £12 million programme was sponsored, to investigate whether BSE was transmitted through embryo transplants or from mother to calf. The experiments collapsed in a shambles when it turned out that most of the experimental cattle were already developing BSE. They had been fed a diet thought to be 'clean' but which was contaminated, as so many others have been, through penny-pinching and illegal recycling.

Science is crucial to our survival, and an understanding of its workings underpins our cultural awareness. The democratization of science, so that it becomes closer to the aspirations of people and understood by everyone, is long overdue. Politicians will openly claim an ignorance of science in a good-humoured and open fashion. They would never admit they could not tell one Brontë sister from another, or could not tell Mozart from Shostakovich; yet few could draw a virus or recognize a cell.

This is serious ignorance. It could now be costing us lives.

12

STARTING OVER

Many voices in the BSE debate have wished we could return to 1980. Could we start to make meat and bone-meal again in the same way that it used to be produced? Would that make it safe again? The idea is attractive, but does not stand up to scrutiny. The traditional fat market collapsed in 1980, and there is no reason to believe that it could ever be reinstated. There are cheaper fat substitutes available. The old processing method, centred on extraction of the fat, was a batch process and costly to use. Modern methods are continuous for long periods, and are far more efficient.

Our current knowledge about the resilience of the BSE agent does not suggest it would necessarily be killed by the rendering process. It is certainly controlled by it, but some could still come through the heat. We also have the problem of supervision and control. For all the regulations on slaughterhouses, we know that about half of them have not been following the rules. In the modern era it would be impossible to make sure that meat and bone-meal from BSE-infected carcases was ever completely safe.

One way to rethink the production of beef would be to separate entirely meat production from the dairy business. All male calves need to have a personal passport, the CID form, which is how farmers apply for subsidies. These are not issued to heifers, so the female members of the cattle population would be handled by a separate system. If the meat industry were restricted to animals bearing the CID passport, then no dairy animals would ever go to slaughter for food. Cows are identified by ear tags, and a central registry could record which were infected, and where they were.

Beef cattle are mainly raised on grass, hay and silage, and have a far lower chance of contracting BSE. It is said that only 15 per cent of beef herds have ever had one or more cases of BSE, compared with half the dairy herds in Britain. One reason for that is earlier slaughter, but another is that these cattle are often fed on vegetation rather than supplements. Over large areas of England, such as the West Country, virtually every herd of dairy cattle has now had at least one case. Raising beef cattle purely for their meat could make a lot of sense. Rather than crossing dairy cattle with beef bulls we'd restrict the breeding to milk breeds and keep the cows solely for dairy.

Although they do not have a very good reputation, the bulls of the beef breeds are a manageable lot. Even the gigantic males, like an Aberdeen Angus bull or a Hereford, have an essentially quiet and placid nature. Farmers know that it is the males of the milk herds, like Friesians, which cause most trouble. Jersey bulls can be very dangerous, for all their placid appearance. We could put dairy cows to dairy bulls, and slaughter any male calves that result. In this way we'd be producing dairy cattle exclusively for milk, and could maintain that principle until BSE was no more. We could continue the supply of milk to the retail markets. Old cows would be slaughtered and incinerated.

Meanwhile the beef business would rely on vegetable and cereal feeds for all their cattle, and there would be no opportunity for an infection to arise. In this way the farms could maintain their present herds, and the food supply would be kept clear of suspect carcases. Quality meat should be at a premium. Old dairy cattle have long been used to produce cheap meat, though you are not likely to see the meat labelled as such in the store. Supermarkets are always trying to drive down costs, and there is a continuing pressure to do things at a bargain price. Our local butcher raises cattle especially for beef on his own smallholding, and never cut his price even at the height of the scare. He could not afford to, because his costings are all controlled. Everyone knows the quality of the meat, so there was no perceived risk from BSE. Britain could adopt a policy of maintaining herds specifically for beef, and separate herds for milk. In this way, the old milk cows would no longer be sold for low-quality meat. We might be able to restore confidence in the quality of the beef.

Confidence is crucial. At the present time, financial institutions do not trust the future for cattle farmers. They are freezing overdrafts promised in happier times and some are refusing to advance the money for a farmer to purchase a new tractor. The restriction on selling cattle has come at a disastrous time for farmers. The arrival of spring in 1996 was greatly delayed (in some areas growth was two months behind) because of a stationary anti-cyclone hovering over Scandinavia. The lack of spring growth in the meadows meant there was no home-grown feed for the stock. It costs £30 per week to feed an animal, and beef farms expect to turn out their cattle to grass in early spring. The lack of growth in 1996 meant that farmers had to buy in supplies to support animals who might be worthless. The competition for feed caused a rise in prices.

April is a time for the payment of farm rents, and cattle farmers had been planning to sell cattle on a set timetable to bring money at that crucial time. The indecision meant that cattle could not be sold at economic rates. Those that could be sold on a subsidized basis brought a financial loss in real terms. This appalling situation continues to inflict hardship on both farmers and their animals.

How old is Recycling?

Farmers have always given scraps to their animals. This is part of the ancient concept of recycling which has become more popular in recent years. Many farm animals eat the oddest things if left to their own devices. I have seen a boar kill and eat an old cockerel in a farmyard. I've watched sheep nibble decorously at fresh placenta in a field. Goats will eat banknotes and ham sandwiches, given half a chance. As we have seen (Chapter 7), cows actually digest animal protein from their herbivorous diet.

Farm animals have probably been fed animal wastes since ancient times. That's why there was a duck-pond on a farm, or at the heart of a village. Small waste scraps were thrown into the water and nourished the pond-life within. The end of the process was the vegetation and the worms which the ducks would eat. As the ducks were consumed, so was the waste that had originally been thrown into the pond. The traditional song about Ilkley Moor portrays the process in prose: the dead body of the subject of the song is destined to be consumed by worms, which will be eaten by ducks, and – when the ducks have been roasted and consumed – 'we will have etten thee'.

Many centuries ago the remains of a carcase were recycled in a manner which reminds us of current practices. After the meat was removed the remains would be boiled down to make a jelly (the liquid was rich in gelatine) and fat would rise to the surface where it set hard on cooling. Part of this became lard, the heavy fat was used in tallow factories to make candles, and the remains were broken up and mixed with cattle and pig food. The notion of animals foraging for grass in the summer sun is attractive, and it is still a common sight, but half the year provides no grass at all and for these bleak months such food reserves have been an important protein supplement.

The Industrialization of Feed Production

As industrialization came to farming, the process of rendering down carcase waste became mechanized. The traditional method was based on the batch processing of a single load of carcases. The waste was chopped into four-inch (10 cm) pieces and heated in a large chamber. The temperature was raised above the boiling-point of water to give a chamber that was at 102-150°C. In some plants the waste was heated up to the working temperature and then discharged; in others it was held at the high temperature and cooked under pressure for up to half an hour. The resulting cooked matter was then cooled and broken down for processing into meal. The fat which remained in the meat was removed by organic solvents by heating to 70°C for 8 hours. The remains were then subjected to superheated steam for 15–30 minutes to remove the solvent for recycling. As we have seen, the risks of handling solvents, coupled with the falling value of the recovered fat, put an end to this practice.

Continuous process came into use after the Second World War. Several different processes were developed. Most of them chopped the waste into scraps an inch or so (3 cms) across. These were heated to a temperature up to 145°C and processed for about an hour. There was considerable variation, however; the Southwood report of 1989 found that one make of drier used temperatures that ranged between 80–145°C. The material took over two hours to pass through, on average, and it was at the maximum temperature for over half an hour.

A new system came into use which separated the cooking and drying functions. The raw material was minced and then raised to 95°C for up to seven minutes. Two processes were offered for the cooked waste. In one system it was dried in batches by being heated to 120–130°C. In the other the product was heated to 800–900°C in a blast of hot air and was then finished off at 110°C.

The type which came to prominence was the Carver-Greenfield processing system. This became the main replacement for the pressurized batch processing machines. The Southwood report set out the operating parameters: waste was heated to 104–123°C and maintained at the raised temperature for fifteen minutes. The entire processing time lasted half an hour or more. Those temperatures do not seem high enough to guarantee sterility even considering conventional pathogens. Reports were published that in 1985 and 1993 the Monopolies and Mergers Commission reprimanded the company for offering inflated prices for carcases in order to exclude competitors.

The immediate conclusion is that the processes varied greatly in terms of the temperature applied. The system of heating to almost a thousand degrees must be a candidate for total sterilization, even from BSE agent, but the use of temperatures around boiling-point would be unlikely to sterilize the product. The pressurized batch systems had been in use for many years. There were few proper controls, and there can be little doubt that proper sterility could not be guaranteed.

The potential hazards had been recognized for years. The Royal Commission on Environmental Pollution published a report in 1979 which remarked: 'The major problem encountered in this recycling process is the risk of transmitting disease-bearing pathogens to stock and thence to humans.'

Protein feed supplements are most often fed to dairy cattle. Many beef farmers make up their own coarse mix for their cattle, much as their forebears have done for centuries. They know how to adjust it, to fit in with what else is available, and the cattle prefer a consistent and predictable feed. A mix of flaked maize and barley is the basis of a nourishing diet from which there is no chance of contracting BSE. The protein supplement that is fed to dairy cows is a product that has been around for a long time. Once it was made with fish-meal, until that became too costly. It comes in bags with little to indicate what lies within. The farmer has to be content with a label that gives the analysis in terms of protein, carbohydrate, fat and ash content. The raw material used by the miller changes with prices. But a farmer used to buying feed at, say, £120–130 per tonne is not likely to suddenly pay more without good reason.

Calling in the Subsidy

The question of subsidy needs to be addressed. It is absurd that we offer such enormous subsidies to farmers. There are local builders, a cinema proprietor, a village shop and an electrician, all of whom could benefit from a little advice and from some financial support when times are hard. None of them is eligible for European support. Yet local farmers can set aside land and receive large payments in the process.

The baron farmers bank six-figure cheques, often for

relatively little effort. They don't like the system any more than the rest of the community, but nobody can blame them for taking full advantage of the way the rules have been drawn. Farming is still the biggest industry of all, and farmers themselves are traditionally conservative voters. It is hardly likely that current governments will vote to do away with such largesse.

In the dairy business the quota system holds sway. There are farmers who buy and sell quotas like a commercial commodity. None of this helps newcomers to the scene, and the future of farming is bleak as long as we tolerate such an absurd system in the biggest business in Britain. We say this is the free market, but the tight controls on this gigantic enterprise are scarcely more rational than anything we used to see in the communist countries.

We urgently need to reconsider the future direction farming can take. The cowmen are themselves a dying breed. Traditional farms run sixty or eighty cattle and have a cowman who is devoted to the task. He knows them all, understands their foibles, and watches out for their welfare. Modern farms (notably in the north-west of Britain) often feature units with 400 cattle or even more. The manager tends to know when he comes to the office, and when he leaves. The twenty-four-hour commitment of the traditional cowman is lost in this big-business attitude. Vets cease to be caring for individual animals, and find they make more and more of their money merely by selling drugs and treatments for the animals.

The financial problems faced by farmers at the present time are serious. Farmers are less willing to call out their vet if there is a difficult birth on the farm, which can be costly in the long run. The illicit burial of cattle, always a potential source of public health hazard, is also set to increase in a situation like this.

The Farmer's Extended Family

No-one should overlook the sense of loss felt by farmers in the present situation. Many of them live and work on family farms that go back generations. They know each animal, care for them, regard them almost as part of an extended family. Earlier in the century the great-grandparents probably raised shorthorns on the farm. After the Second World War the grandparents very likely turned to Friesians, and since then a modern generation will have moved towards Charolais cattle. Each farm has its own sense of tradition, and the prospect of all cattle over a given age being destroyed – even those from healthy, grass-fed herds – has had many farmers contemplating suicide, if not homicide.

Could discarded carcases be used for pet food? Incineration is the only safe and sure way of disposing of the agent for good, and any use in pet food has to be given careful consideration before it is ever permitted. Of the seventy-one cases of feline spongiform encephalopathy recorded so far, all seem to stem from contaminated pet food. This is a very small number of cases given the entire feline population of Britain, but is a great tragedy for the families who have lost their pets. Dogs have not shown susceptibility to the agent, and the marketing of suspect carcases in dog food is bound to be proposed. Incineration must remain the preferred option. We have to do all we can to eliminate the agent from existence, as far as is humanly possible.

One of the major beef-producing nations is the USA, and so far not a single case of BSE has been reported from United States farms. There has been just one case in Canada. That does not mean that the topic is of little interest in North America. Professor Hugh Lewis is an expatriate Welshman who is now Dean at the Veterinary School of Purdue University, at West Lafayette, Indiana.

He runs a phone-in enquiry line for veterinarians with scientific questions. 'At the present time, 80 per cent of our enquiries concern BSE,' he said in April 1996. There is a coast-to-coast watch for cattle imported into the USA from Britain during the at-risk years.

Country	Total BSE cases
Britain	161,700
Switzerland	206
Ireland	123
Portugal	31
France	13
Germany	4
Italy	2
Oman	2
Canada	1
Denmark	1
Falklands	1

Table 14: Which countries have BSE?

In terms of the incidence of BSE in the national herd, Switzerland is second to Britain in the league table. This statistic produced some comment early on, because Switzerland is free from scrapie and has lush pastureland in abundance. The reason lies in the source of the protein supplements sold in Switzerland. Between 1985–1990, 22 per cent of their meat and bone-meal was imported into Switzerland from Britain.

Much of the talk of the purity of foreign beef can be deceptive. The regulations covering the production of meat apply across the whole of Europe, it's true, but we are one of the countries which largely put them into operation. In some of the Mediterranean lands there is a fine tradition of defying bureaucracy, and the health standards of the meat that results does not meet British requirements. Not only that, but large numbers of European farms have had feed and animals from Britain. We have exported huge amounts of feedstuffs containing contaminated meal, and have exported tonnes of bonemeal itself to other nations. Many thousand head of cattle have been exported to countries across Europe from BSE-infected herds. As we bring beef in from outside, we must be buying back some of the stock we exported.

The number of recorded cases does not necessarily reflect reality, for farmers in some nations are disinclined to report in when a cow goes sick. The current incidence is related to the export of meal (and cattle) from Britain. But the problem is now, regrettably, a European one. Little wonder Egypt has decided to ban all imports of European cattle, not merely those from the UK.

We now have a strange situation. There are unprecedented controls on British beef, which prevent its export in any form. We are going to see strong action taken to move towards the elimination of BSE from the national herd, and this moves us closer to a BSE-free era. To cover any shortfall, or to ward against a drop in sales, imported beef is now being touted as the safer alternative. The result may be to expose us to new risks.

We may end up with the only guaranteed BSE-free beef in Europe. The meat being imported in the interests of public confidence is already presenting an increased risk from containing antibiotics and growth hormones – together with the agent of BSE that had originally been unwittingly exported from British shores. Foreign beef is not necessarily safe beef. We would do well to remember that.

13

WHERE DID BSE COME FROM?

Here we are on firm ground. Everyone seems agreed about the original source: it came from scrapie in unsterilized cattle feed. Scrapie used to infect sheep and now it infects cattle as well. So that's easily explained.

It may be easy, but I believe it may be wrong.

There is evidence to suggest that BSE has been around for longer than the authorities admit. In addition, the BSE agent may not have come from scrapie crossing the species barrier. There have been references to scrapie in cows for many years. The earliest published case was in France, where in 1829 a naturalist named Berger compiled an account of a disease which is very like today's reports of BSE. There have been rumours of scrapie in oxen from before the First World War in the English Lake District. Several reports have circulated of cases of scrapie in cattle seen in Cornwall years ago, and of cows with abnormal behaviour in southern England. When an occasional case is reported, it is easy to overlook it. In this way it is possible we have failed to recognize what may be an important syndrome.

As an example, take the recollections of Andrew Biggs,

a West Country veterinary surgeon. 'I well remember going to see a cow at one of the farms in the practice, when I was a very young vet,' he says. 'The cow had the staggers, caused by hypomagnesaemia, too little magnesium in the body. She had fallen down, and I had to give her barbiturates to prevent her having fits. I'm afraid she was very ill by the time I got there, and she never recovered.

'At the time, nobody would have thought of BSE. It was still unknown. But many years later a colleague of mine was called to a farm, to look at a cow with a similar condition, milk fever. That's due to too little calcium in the blood, hypocalcaemia. She had collapsed, and he gave her the injection that soon had her up on her feet again. A couple of weeks later I was called to see the same cow. She had collapsed once more. I gave her the calcium treatment, but this time she didn't recover as I expected. I told the farmer that she looked a bit odd, and he told me that's what my colleague had remarked two weeks earlier. This time the cow did not improve. This was in the era of BSE, so we called in the Ministry vet and indeed she was a victim of the disease. But I sometimes wonder how many cases in the past which didn't get better were actually BSE all the while. It is perfectly possible it did exist, in small numbers.'

BSE – an Alternative View

There is a possible alternative source of the present BSE outbreak. The greatest problem posed by the conventional view is the way in which an infection confined to sheep for centuries could suddenly take to infecting cows. If the agent has long existed in cattle, then we do not need to speculate on how an agent can spread from one ruminant species to another. BSE could be an ancient disease of cattle, then this puzzling phenomenon would not be a necessary part of the argument.

The molecular studies of the disease provide support from a different angle. If BSE arose from incompletely sterilized carcases infected with scrapie, then you might expect to see several strains of BSE just as there are of scrapie. Analysis of the infection shows that all the specimens isolated so far are identical. There are a great many strains of scrapie known, but each isolate of BSE is the same. There can be only one conclusion: the BSE agent arose from one case, and this single case has given rise to every BSE infection since.

Research reported from Iowa on 11 April 1996 claimed that the experimental administration of sheep scrapie into calves certainly produced a lethal disease, but not BSE. It was quickly said that this would make a ban on infected feed irrelevant. Yet there are objections. One obvious explanation would be that the wrong type of strain was used. But there is another view, namely that the original agent arose, not in sheep, *but in cows.*

The news media have reported extensively on the way that discarded and sub-standard sheep carcases have been used as a protein source to make meal destined for cattle feed. What has not been emphasized is that sub-standard *cattle* carcases have also been recycled in exactly the same manner. Cattle fed on protein supplement over the years have probably consumed more feed made from bovine carcases than from sheep. One of the critics of the system has said that he was alerted to the fact that cows were being fed recycled cattle protein when he first visited a rendering plant and watched how the protein supplement was produced. 'We were actually recycling cattle to cattle,' he wrote. 'To me it's cannibalism. That was a big mistake.' Interestingly, this visit to an animal feed factory was made in the early 1970s. If it was a mistake, it was fifteen years before anything happened. This must suggest that it was not the simple act of recycling which alone was the problem. There must surely have been a new factor which suddenly came into play.

We have seen that there is not a *prima facie* reason against adding an animal protein supplement, provided it is safely prepared and is scientifically incorporated into a balanced feed. There is a far more reasonable explanation for the origins of the outbreak in 1985. Let us assume that BSE has always existed in cattle. It is not a contagious disease. The chances of it being spread are low. How it could survive from one generation is largely a mystery, but it would presumably pass along in cattle as scrapie passes in sheep.

Whenever an infected cattle carcase had come to the rendering plant in the past, the processing would have inactivated the agent. From 1982, however, that all changed. New processing plants involved lower processing temperatures. From this date on, there was an added possibility for an infection to survive. We could suppose that a carcase already infected with BSE was sent to the plant. The protein product was incorporated into cattle feed. From that moment on the agent had a new route for transmission. Once cattle began to become ill with the disease (remember that the first known case arose three years later) their discarded carcases might be noted as unfit for human consumption and sent to the rendering plant for processing into feed. As soon as that had happened, the infection in the feed was being returned in diseased carcases and an epidemic was set to start.

To me, this view makes far more sense in many ways. Catching BSE from scrapie is hard to conceive, but catching BSE from a cattle carcase already infected with this agent is much easier to envisage. The recycling of carcases through feed means that cattle were contracting the disease from the remains of infected cattle, and not from the related disease in sheep.

There is an even more bizarre prospect. Sheep fed on a BSE-contaminated diet develop what looks like scrapie, but when the agent is injected into mice they develop the signs, *not* of scrapie, but of BSE. It is just possible that sheep may have caught BSE from contaminated feed, and if so there may now be *two* spongy-brain diseases existing in the sheep population. There are currently 20 million sheep in Britain, worth £1.2 billion a year to the farmers. Were sheep offal to be banned as a precaution there would be extensive repercussions. There would be no more Scottish haggis, for a start.

It remains possible that the outbreak comes from other sources and is not connected with meal. In one survey, scientists from the Ministry of Agriculture, Fisheries and Food compared figures from herds that were fed concentrate, with those that had apparently never eaten this feed. In one survey they found that 98.6 per cent of BSE-positive herds had eaten concentrate, whilst 97.6 per cent of herds free of BSE had apparently done so. In one sample of 42 BSE-negative herds, 41 were said to have eaten concentrate.

Is there any evidence that other forms of spongy-brain disease existed in the past? Perhaps the cat disease FSE is an old condition which we are only recognizing after the sudden surge of interest. There are many collections of microscope slides made from animal specimens, and these have been searched. There are no signs of any cat brain sections showing FSE dated earlier than the era of contaminated pet food. It truly seems to be a new disease, and may well have been contracted from pet food made with contaminated carcases.

The main question centres on the young human victims of the disease. If cattle with BSE gave rise to the recycling of infection, then some sensation-seeking scientist is bound to suggest that human remains (from a victim of CJD) were once sold to a pie-manufacturer. If the rumour starts, don't believe it. CJD contamination infects other people with CJD, not with the strain of kuru we have witnessed in the new disease. The paper on this tragic outbreak was published in the *Lancet* in April 1996 and showed that the symptoms were different from those of CJD, and there is a good case to be made that this is the wrong name for the disease (Chapter 8).

How new is it? Anecdotal evidence suggests that there have been young victims in the past. They have perhaps been diagnosed as suffering from Alzheimer's disease, and noted as particularly young victims of the condition. A syndrome only appears when you see a significant number of people with virtually identical signs and symptoms, and it is possible that isolated cases have always occurred, but have never been brought to a common focus in the past because there was no national research programme to seek them out.

The sensible conclusion at this stage is that these are cases of BSE transferred to humans. It is sensible because it heightens official concern, and will encourage the Government to take a long-term view of the problem. If this helps the eradication of BSE (as we have already seen the elimination of the smallpox virus) it can only be for the good. However, there is still no scientific reason to suppose that these new cases arose from infected beef. A search of museum specimens of brain tissue, often preserved in the form of sections mounted on microscope slides, suggests that the disease may have been in existence for years.

A survey of existing brain sections could reveal whether there are such patients from the past. One such slide museum is the Corsellis collection at Runwell Hospital, Essex. This has been examined, together with slides in other collections. Dr Gareth Roberts of the pharmaceutical company Smith Kline Beecham has looked at 8,000 brain sections and narrowed them down to 1,100 from patients who had died of dementia. Of these, he found microscopical evidence of CJD in nineteen slides. Only eleven of those had been diagnosed during life, for the remaining eight had not been recognized. In this sample, 40 per cent of the cases had been missed during life. One died in 1980 aged forty, another in 1978 aged forty-eight.

This may mean that there has been consistent under-reporting of these diseases for years. Dr Roberts is of no doubt that the 'new' form of spongy-brain disease has been around for many years. Most of these cases have been diagnosed as Alzheimer's of the young. There have been many strange cases over the years, which psychiatrists are unable to identify and which end in the death of the patient. Dr Roberts says, 'Perhaps the people in Edinburgh have suddenly discovered what we have already seen.' His joint paper was published in *Neurodegeneration* in December 1995. That was the same month in which Peter Martin, the *Mail on Sunday* journalist, was told by the Government that his allegation that there were young victims was 'misleading and untrue'.

The censorship of open discussion by the British government has been an international disgrace. The leading scientific journal *Nature* **380:** 370 on 4 April 1996 reports that the Edinburgh group who investigated the new cases was due to present a report on the epidemiology of CJD in Britain at an international conference of spongiform encephalopathies in Paris. When the news of the paper in the *Lancet* was about to break, the team was recalled to Britain by the UK government and were not able to present their findings.

Olivier Robain, the leading authority on prions in Paris, asked pointedly, 'Was this censorship by the British government?' The Director-General of INSERM, the French biomedical research agency, said that this 'unacceptable' behaviour had 'triggered reactions of panic'. Professor Hans-Dieter Klenk, the senior virologist at Marburg University, says the action 'fanned public hysteria'. In Switzerland, the Director of the Institute of Molecular Biology in Zurich, Professor Charles Weissmann, contrasted the way the British government told the public there was never any risk, yet simultaneously warned farmers and slaughterhouse staff that they should be 'very careful how you handle the cattle and the meat'.

It has now been confirmed that there are cases of the new strain of human spongy-brain disease in other countries. Two have been reported from Germany. In France a young man of twenty-seven who died in Lyons in January has now been confirmed as a victim of the new strain. Jean-François Girard, Director General of Health in France, said this means the problem is now a European one.

Though the fact was not been reported in the English language press, there have also been two cases in the Netherlands. The younger one, from the town of Houten, died of the disease aged thirty-two. One Dutch professor says, ' The general idea here is that it is all the fault of the British for being inefficient in this as other things. Meat in general, and beef in particular, have suffered spectacular falls in sales. At the university canteen, piles of nicely underdone beef slices were left unsold at the end of the day. All the shops have notices emphasizing *Slechts Hollands vlees* (only Dutch meat) or *Geen buitenlandse produkten* (no foreign produce).'

Which Animals are Sick?

The experience of the British farming community still throws up puzzles for science. Not every at-risk animal contracts the disease. Angus and Jean Campbell farm in the Kent village of Pluckley. They fed cattle-cake to all their cows. Four calves of one of their cows contracted BSE in autumn 1991. All died. The mother of these calves, who had eaten even more of the supplement, remained healthy.

There are many rumours about the extent of BSE in the differing breeds of cattle. Several people have told me within the last week that they eat Aberdeen Angus beef, since the butchers assure them that the breed has never has a case of BSE. That's not so. The April 1996 total of cases in the Angus herds was 1,349.

Breed	Cases	Breed	Cases
Angus	1,349	Ankole	2
Ayrshire	1,679	Bazadaise	1
Bel Gal	2	Belgian Blue	184
Black Her	7	Black Limousin	1
Black d'Aquitaine	133	Blue Grey	13
Blue Roan	3	British White	51
Brown Swiss	52	Canadian Angus	3
Canadian Guernsey	1	Charolais	952
Chianina	4	Devon	130
Dexter	0	Dutch Holstein	1
Friesian	134,710	Galloway	27
Gelbveih	33	Gloucester	2
Guernsey	1,452	Hereford	8,395
Highland	18	Irish Moiled	0
Jersey	1,467	Kerry	0
Limousin	2,496	Lincoln Red	12

Breed	Cases	Breed	Cases
Longhorn	7	Luing	4
Marchigiana	2	Meuse Rhine Issel	28
Murray Grey	53	Normandy	2
North Devon	47	Piedmontese	8
Red Friesian	277	Red Holstein	8
Red Poll	36	Romagnola	6
Saler	8	Shorthorn	349
Simmenthal	2,250	South Devon	124
South Down	1	Sussex	133
Welsh Black	83	White Park	2
Others	2,526		
		TOTAL	159,134

Table 15: Cattle Breeds affected to April 1996

This list contains a most intriguing piece of evidence for the ability of some breeds to resist, or perhaps even to hide, an infection. Just three breeds show a zero score in the above table. They are the Irish Moiled, the Kerry and the Dexter. All are descended from the Bronze Age cattle. They are hardy, small animals. There is no doubt that all of them have been fed supplementary rations containing the same infected meal as all the other breeds.

To date, none of them has gone down with BSE. This may be because they are able to throw off the infection. Does this offer a clue as to how we can study resistance to BSE? Can it reveal that ancient cattle were exposed to the agent and evolved means to deal with it – which later breeds have lost? Time will tell. At the present, this is another aspect of the mystery.

14

WHAT CAUSES A SPONGY BRAIN?

There have been many theories on the cause of spongy-brain disease. As is the way with science, the nature of the latest theory says a lot about the current fashions in scientific research. When people in the past first put forward ideas about a strange, new infective principle (which is what we currently believe) they were ridiculed. We rarely stop to consider why a specific theme underpins a new scientific theory, but it has much to do with the latest trends and the need to be fashionable. Ideas in science rise and fall like discs in the pop charts, and for surprisingly similar reasons.

Slow Viruses

The 'slow virus' concept of the Icelandic researcher Björn Sigurdsson (Chapter 3) fitted the facts as they were known at the time, but there have been many later theories. Sigurdsson showed that the infections did not spread widely in the body of the animal, but were usually confined to a single organ. The prolonged incubation period of months or decades led to a degenerative disease that was invariably fatal. Those interesting factors gave a sense that the diseases had much in common, but closer scrutiny disproved the idea. They had little in common in terms of the symptoms they caused, and were clearly unrelated diseases in that sense. The speed with which a disease develops was shown to be a property of lots of different viruses, rather than one or two groups; and finally, no virus was ever found for scrapie. There was not even the diagnostic sign of a virus taking hold, namely, the production by the body of the antibodies which protect against an invading germ.

An Imbalanced Diet

There is always a nutritional theory for a disease like spongy-brain. This one argues that the diet of captive animals can lack a vital component, and this could cause the disease. Here the argument centres on α-linoleic acid. In the body this is made into docosahexaenoic acid, which is vital for the brain cells. There is a lot of this kind of compound in vegetable foods, but not in meat protein. The theory argued that, since cattle and the antelopes are all captive, maybe the change of their diet from one rich in vegetable constituents to one containing animal protein had caused the lack of α-linoleic acid, and that led to the spongy brain. Studies of the way the disease spread, and which herds were affected, did not relate the illness to the balance of the diet. Not only that, but there was no evidence that the α-linoleic acid was actually missing from the diet, anyway.

High Nitrogen Fertilizers

Fertilizers are over-used in modern intensive agriculture, and they are regularly the target of suspicion when any new disease comes along. Here there were several theories. The simplest said that the use of fertilizers meant that animals were taking in too much protein from their food. Others said that there was a knock-on effect. The fertilizer increased the release of somatotrophin in the body, which in turn triggered metabolic change which gave rise to spongy-brain disease. I could never quite work out how that was supposed to happen, and in any event the theory did not hold water. For one thing, there were large herds of beef cattle feeding on intensively fertilized vegetation across great areas of the United States, yet not a single case of BSE has yet been reported there. If the fertilizer was to blame, the incidence of BSE would follow the use of fertilizer. Clearly, this was not the case.

Phosphorus Pesticides

One theory which keeps surfacing is that pesticides were to blame. The organophophorus compounds (OPC's) used to protect farm animals from warble fly are the main candidate. The OPC's are dangerous. Farm-workers handling them have to wear protective clothing. Some who have been exposed to the liquids have become very ill. The sickness affects the nervous system, and it takes a time to appear. There is an obvious possibility that, if OPC's cause harm to the nerves, perhaps spongy-brain disease might be caused by them too. The scientific evidence does not back the idea. Many of the cases of spongy-brain disease have had no contact with pesticides. The signs of BSE are not like those of the nerve damage caused by the OPC's. There are areas where OPC's are not used (Guernsey, for example), but where BSE is found. Other nations (like the USA) use plenty of pesticides, but have no BSE. These reasons suggest that the pesticide theory is a non-starter.

Bacteria

Bacteria were highly fashionable for scientific research between the mid 1800s and the mid 1900s. Since then they were displaced in the attention of microbiologists by viruses, which became the high-profile target for research. This has been a mistake. Bacteria remain a crucial area for investigation. For example, ten years ago it was found that stomach ulcers are not caused by stress, by diet, by your job, or by any of the generally accepted causes, but by a germ. The bacterium responsible is *Helicobacter pylori*, and it can be cured in most people by a cocktail of antibiotics. It now seems likely that this bacterium causes stomach cancer as well, so a course of treatment could perhaps reduce the incidence of that major disease. Few doctors have even heard of this important discovery. We are keenly taking antacids, like the proprietary Zantac, adding millions to the coffers of the pharmaceutical industry, where there is a relatively cheap and permanent treatment available. That's how fashion influences public health.

Could these brain diseases also be caused by a neglected bacterium? Some reports have suggested this. A strange organism looking a little like a familiar *Spiroplasma* has been found in brain tissues taken from victims of Creutzfeldt-Jakob disease. Word on the street is that the existence of this organism is not always associated with spongy-brain disease, so it is unlikely to be the cause. It does seem to react in the same way as the prion protein which is at the centre of the current favourite theory when tested in the laboratory, though whether this is the result of the disease or (perhaps) its cause we must wait to see.

A Nerve-cell Theory

Could the disease be a reaction to an escaped fragment of nerve-cell membrane that spreads through the brain? The idea would work like this: a minute fragment of the membrane covering a nerve-cell would escape and start making membrane in places where it shouldn't. Some of these membrane molecules are very resistant to heat and to disinfectant agents, so it is always possible that the agent of BSE and the other diseases arose from a nerve cell. There is very little support for such a theory, and more evidence to substantiate that it might work are what we need next.

Viruses and 'Virinos'

Many of the reports have spoken of the BSE 'virus'. No such thing has been found. Since the slow virus idea was discounted in spongy-brain disease, scientists have been looking for some kind of virus. So far the search has not proved conclusive. In recent years it has been thought that a simplified virus, a 'virino', might be the cause. No-one has produced the evidence to substantiate this theory.

Another fascinating possibility is that there might be a strange tiny virus-like entity with a single strand of DNA. This has been named a 'nemavirus'. Studies with the electron microscope have shown some strange structures which, it is claimed, have three layers. There is an outer layer of protein, a central layer of the single-strand of DNA, and a core within of the prion protein we shall encounter later. The reports suggest that these odd filamentous structures are found only in cases of a spongy-brain disease. Few scientists are convinced, but this idea is still current.

Sperm

In 1990 there was speculation that the agent was transmitted through semen. A farmer in Yorkshire claimed that, although all his cattle had eaten the same feed, the only ones to develop the signs of BSE were those sired by the same bull. The seminal fluid of British bulls (widely used for artificial insemination) was banned by several non-EEC countries because of the possible risk. Australia and New Zealand, with Sweden, Finland and Russia were the first to impose bans on British bull semen. Eighty per cent of British calves are the result of artificial insemination (AI) and the possibility of transmission required investigation. The Central Veterinary Laboratory set about checking semen samples for the infective agent. They had stocks of 850 semen samples, and extensive research was undertaken before the idea of an association between semen and BSE was shelved.

Prions

These are the currently favoured theory. This is still a theory, but there is much evidence to suggest prions could be the cause of the spongy brain. It certainly provides a serious working hypothesis unless and until something better emerges. What does 'prion' stand for? That depends on where you look. One early definition said it was derived from *protease resistant protein*. The most recent description, published in April 1996, said it came from *proteinaceous infectious particle*. I doubt whether the latter etymology makes any sense at all. Every germ is an infectious protein particle, and the point about the prion is that it resists the normal enzymes (proteases) which do attack proteins. That's why prions are hard to destroy.

We all produce prions in normal brain cells. The gene which produces prion protein (known as the PrP gene for short) is also found in other mammals. The prion gene is translated into messenger RNA which assembles the molecules and generates the prions. These are produced in two forms, either as spiral molecules or as pleated sheets. The theory suggests that some forms of prion protein fail to fold properly. They grow at unaccustomed angles, and the result is damage to the brain cells. The

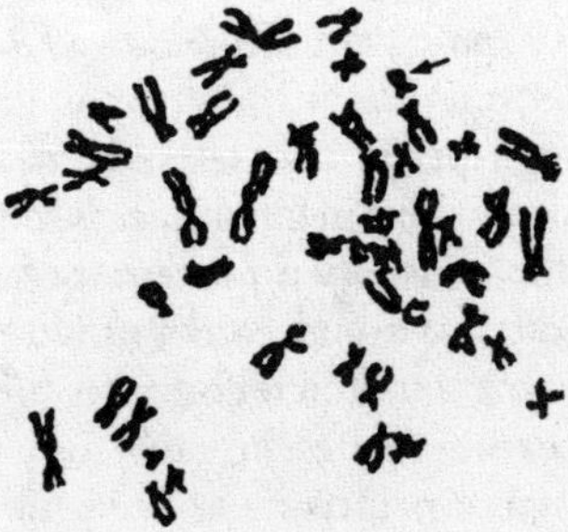

Fig 7: Human chromosomes

The nucleus of a human cell, cultured in a laboratory, arranges its chromosomes together in a layer across the middle of the cell as it prepares to divide in half. At this stage it is possible to squash the cell and study the separate chromosomes. Chromosome number 20 (arrowed, top right) carries the genes that make prion proteins.

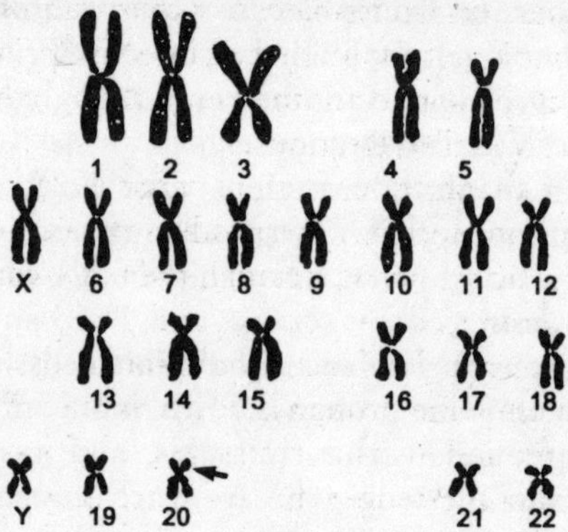

Fig 8: Chromosome map

Photographs of the chromosomes can be sorted out and identified. The X and Y chromosomes are the ones which determine the sex of the individual (XX is a female, XY a male). On the short arm of chromosome 20 (arrowed) lie the prion genes. Mutations of these are now known, and can regulate how a spongy-brain disease will develop.

transmissible spongy-brain diseases seem to come about when an altered prion protein gains access to the cells and starts producing the misshapen protein molecules.

Some forms of disease are already known to be caused by mutations of the gene which codes for prions. There are 23 pairs of chromosomes in each human cell, and the genes which make prions have been located on the short arm of chromosome 20. There are many mutations already known in this area. Many of them are associated with human disease. One mutation has been found in several families with fatal familial insomnia, FFI (Chapter 5). Another, a little further along the chromosome, has been found in three clusters of Creutzfeldt-Jakob disease in Libya, Slovakia and Chile. The fact that CJD has been shown to be infectious in humans (and transmissible to other animals) is a surprising finding. It shows that an infective principle can pass from one person to another, even though the disease itself is not normally infectious.

When conventional infections take hold, the host body usually responds by producing antibodies to attack the invading agent. Though there are some forms of antigen produced by scrapie and BSE, anti-scrapie antibodies are not produced in the infected sheep, and there is no immune response. This makes it hard to detect the disease in its early stages, and has posed a major problem for those who are searching for a quick test for the diseases.

Crystallization

A simpler theory has been put forward. This suggests that the prion protein forms crystals in infected cells, and these cause the disruption we can see. There is already known to be a problem with a β-amyloid in Alzheimer's disease. The result is that plaques of deposits of amyloid, a substance laid down in several diseases, form in the brain tissues. Though that may be the case, no-one denies that in many spongy-brain diseases there are no amyloid deposits. Clearly, the theory would not apply easily to those cases. It does provide an intriguing link between spongy-brain disease and other forms of brain degeneration.

In some ways the prion theory has much in common with this idea of crystallization. A related idea suggests that the misshapen prion protein could act as a key, triggering other molecules to be produced in a similar shape. This has been known as the *molecular chaperon theory*, and it does have much in common with the prion concept.

New forms of Life

One interesting discovery may relate to the spongy-brain diseases, even if it is not itself the cause. A new form of infectious agent has been discovered in fluid taken from the lower part of the human intestine, the ileum. It has been named 'intestinal fluid-dependent organism' (IFDO for short). This is a remarkable new life form. It is unaffected by the same temperatures which scrapie can survive, and is not affected by many of the same disinfectants. It resists nuclear radiation. It is said that these tiny organisms look like the thread-like prions seen in the electron microscope, but they are different from prions in several respects. IFDO's are inactivated by several compounds which don't have any effect on scrapie, including zinc nitrate. However, if IFDO's are incubated with fatty substances, lipoproteins, from then on they aren't affected by zinc nitrate. Nobody knows why, or what they really are.

It is clear that these IFDO's are similar to scrapie in some ways, yet different in others. Most importantly, research into tissue samples from cattle with BSE and sheep with scrapie has not shown any IFDO's. It seems as though they are a potentially important new discovery, but not the cause of spongy-brain disease.

At present, we are learning more about the diseases, but still cannot say exactly what causes them. The proponents of the different theories advance their views, sometimes with the enthusiasm of salesmen, and once in a while acceptability seems to be related to the professionalism of the sales pitch. In an age of competition for grants, when the idea of money is the distant lure, promotion matters as much as objectivity. Scientists are often on short-term contracts these days, and securing the next grant matters above all else. The need to present a convincing grant application has become a science in itself, and in a commercial era it is hard to keep a hold on scientific reality.

When money comes into the equation, scientific truth goes out of the window.

15

THESE ARE THE RISKS

Let us put matters into perspective. We will start by assuming that the new tragic young victims of spongy-brain disease contracted the illness from eating beef. They have been reported over two years. That gives an annual rate of six per year. The population of Britain is 58 million, of which perhaps half eat beef. This means that the chances of having contracted the disease is about one in five million. To the people involved, and statisticians would do well to remember this, it is a terrible and debilitating end. The tragedy to the families is utterly unimaginable, and the sense that the loss could have been prevented by sensible action makes matters far worse.

Living will always surround all of us with risk. We stay alive on the basis of a running lottery which picks us off more or less at random. We have a chance to load the dice in our favour, but although that can bias some of the chances it cannot reduce them to zero. Other hazards are worth setting into context. Half the British population, early each Saturday evening, believe they are going to win the National Lottery that night. I find it embarrassing to admit, having appeared on the BBC programme *National*

Lottery Live as their 'guest pundit', but I have even felt that sense of anticipation personally. The chance of winning the jackpot is one in fourteen million. There's a one in five million chance of being struck by lightning over the next two years, or of being killed in a railway accident within the next month. If you are forty, then the chance of dying within a year from natural causes is already more than one in a thousand, and the odds keep shortening as time ticks by.

Event	Chance of one in
Struck by lightning	10,000,000
Beef risk (as above)	5,000,000
Death in railway accident	500,000
Being murdered	100,000
Dying in domestic accident	26,000
Dying in road accident	8,000
Death through influenza	5,000
Natural causes, middle-aged	850
Smoking 10 cigarettes a day	200

Table 16: Risks of death during the next twelve months

These statistics do not presuppose that there is no further hazard from spongy-brain disease in humans. They simply set into context the risks we daily take for granted. The tragic youngsters who died of spongy-brain disease stood a chance more than 600 times bigger if they travelled by car, and if you include serious injury on the roads and disfigurement for life the chances are more than 1,000 times bigger. We are certain that stress and undue anxiety are themselves a predisposition to morbidity, and it would not be right to make yourself ill with fear for the future on little account. There is a ten times greater chance of dying in a railway accident next year, yet I do not imagine that will prevent people from travelling by rail.

Where do you turn for advice if you wish to reduce your risks? You might take advice from acknowledged scientific authorities. The highest scientific authority in Britain is the Royal Society of London, which has acted as the repository for scientific wisdom for more than three centuries. They have arbitrated over the unravelling of science, from the grace and intellectualism of natural philosophy to the modern technocracy where few have the broad mind that science truly entails. A casualty of the great tradition has been the presentation of scientific ideas clearly and openly to the public. One of their most important early books, Robert Hooke's *Micrographia* of 1665, was the first monumental work on the microscope, and was directed straight at the public. It makes a timely comparison with their latest document, a summary of knowledge on BSE. In the eleven paragraphs of this statement, there are roughly the same number of errors.

'Many people,' says the opening sentence, 'rightly looked to the scientific community for guidance about bovine spongiform encephalopathy (BSE) and its possible connection with Creutzfeldt-Jakob disease (CJD).' They may look but there is little to satisfy that natural desire in this well-intentioned paper. 'The human form [of SE] is CJD,' they say, heedless of kuru and fatal familial insomnia. 'The infectious agents . . . are prions,' claims the document, evading the need to explain that there are other possible explanations. 'BSE was first seen in 1986,' readers are assured, although there are indications that earlier cases were observed.

The document extols the importance of the interplay between scientific understanding and public perceptions whilst abandoning the principles: 'BSE has been found to infect other species,' it states, calmly, and then adds, 'it must therefore be possible that BSE could infect humans.' Friends of the Royal Society will sigh indulgently at this exemplar of the chasm between science and the public. The sceptic will snort and say, '*Now* they tell us.'

In science, hindsight can be more useful in proving you were right than any grant.

Outbreak of a New Disease

Spongy-brain diseases are increasing. A century ago the only one we knew was scrapie, common in sheep. Three-quarters of a century ago we were discovering there was a rare disease in humans, comparable in some ways to scrapie, called Creutzfeldt-Jakob disease. The risk of suffering from classical CJD is about one in a million. Half a century ago we added kuru to the list. This came from cannibalism, and claimed the lives of one person in a hundred each year. That is a devastating burden on any society (it is about the same as the deaths among heavy cigarette-smokers).

Though we do not know for sure that the recent cases in young Britons are the result of consuming contaminated offal, the association is a reasonable one. The fact that we can say so is in stark contrast to the Government's assurances that beef was definitely perfectly safe, during the years that science was waving a warning finger. If so, the cases could be the tip of a growing problem. Sir Richard Southwood, the Vice-Chancellor of Oxford who chaired the early enquiries into BSE and people, has even said that the number at risk could be in the millions.

Although the regulations have called for the banning of offal from the food supply, there is insufficient training and too little money to do the job properly. There is now provision for vets to be on duty in slaughterhouses. This is a monotonous task, and most British vets have not found it a productive way to spend their days. As a result, vets from anywhere in the European Union have been brought in to fulfil the task. Some of them are not much good.

The new scheme was set up in January 1995 to replace the old local authority inspectors. It was called the Meat Hygiene Service. In practice it has failed. Agency vets have been brought in to provide the statutory personnel, but abattoir managers say that many of them have hardly any knowledge of English, are rarely seen to be doing the job properly, and do not always supervise the removal of condemned offal as they are required to do. The abattoirs have been informed that the previous hourly pay rate of £15 has more than doubled to £35 per hour, and managers say that the additional money is not bringing the service expected. Many of the agency vets have only had experience of domestic dogs and cats.

We thus have a system where specified offal is meant to be kept out of the food supply. Official statements reassure the public because of the new restrictions – but the reality is that the supervision is lacking and the system is unreliable. If the 48 per cent failure rate is still the norm, then the system has only been half effective. That is not enough to restore public confidence, and will do nothing to assist the restoration of the trade in British beef and its products. Some farmers and dealers have been falsifying records in order to sell meat from suspect cattle as though they were certified BSE-free. In spot checks of abattoirs, there were at least twenty-one instances where spinal cord (possibly infected with BSE agent) had not been discarded as the regulations require.

Planning and Risk

Some official actions have exposed us all to greater risks than need have been the case. No specialists in infectious spongy-brain diseases were brought into the committees at the outset. There were no fiscal incentives to prevent the dissemination of infected cattle, and no attempt to stop breeding in infected herds. It was widely believed that cattle would be the final host for the virus, whilst it was being agreed that scrapie had jumped to one new species already. The amount of research into transmissibility is still far too small, and it remains difficult to understand why the export of infected cattle (and contaminated feed) went on for so long.

The tool we use to reduce all risks is knowledge. Knowledge comes from enquiry and experience. At this very moment, Western governments are considering ways to hive off academic research and put it in the hands of private enterprise. Individual research, fired by the spark of fascination for the truth, is the key to all scientific enquiry. In that sense, private science is real science. But the commercial privatization of science is a trap. Market-driven research, aimed at wealth creation, funds programmes where there is profit in view. We need something else to fund knowledge creation! Research into scrapie was always driven by curiosity, and never by a quest for profit. No private organization would have poured millions into something so speculative, yet scientific research into scrapie now turns out to have been vital.

Another way to reduce risk is to regulate affairs to limit the chances of infection. Merely introducing regulations is never enough. If we are to reduce individual risks, then we need to see they are carried out. The Treasury needs to set funds aside for this very task. What of the feed still in the pipeline? Government decrees ban food, which makes it unlawful to use it from that moment on. But many farmers, whether they are raising cattle or trout, are prudent enough to have stocks in store. This represents hundreds of pounds tied up in unusable stock. They have bought it in only because the Government has given assurances that it's safe to use.

Who is going to buy it back and safely dispose of it? Are farmers going to use it, if they cannot afford to absorb the loss? I would guess that much of this contaminated feed is going to be fed to animals, ban or no ban. The losers should be offered compensation by the Treasury. Public consumers are put at additional risk, and this must be stopped.

Since the first research on mad cow disease, the agent has been found to concentrate itself in the central nervous system. Experiments to transmit the agent from muscle tissue, red meat, have not been successful. Those who have consumed steak are likely to be unaffected by the agent of spongy-brain disease. The greatest risk is in people who have eaten the mix of waste matter – brain, spinal cord and the rest – which goes to help bulk out cheap products. The most vulnerable members of society are likely to be victims.

The 'No-risk' Strategy

One crucial question was posed to me, as I was compiling this section. It was this: how could one reduce *all* risks from food to an absolute minimum? Vegetables, we have discovered, are naturally rich in potentially poisonous compounds. Grilled meat brings risks from heart attacks and cancer. Sometimes the diet seems as potent as an agent for disease as it is an arbiter of health. The no-risk stratagem doesn't exist. I speculated on the most innocuous situation imaginable, and envisaged staying in bed, subsisting on watercress and lightly boiled eggs whilst drinking nothing but water.

Think it through. The egg is rich in cholesterol, and (if lightly boiled) it may give you *Salmonella*. The watercress would have to be cooked, to ensure there was no risk from liver-fluke. The water might well be high in nitrates, and could pass on *Cryptosporidium* which is hard to identify and impossible to cure. Might you give up food altogether? Even that is no answer. Staying in bed brings the risk from a deep-vein thrombosis or (if that eludes you) there is always hypostatic pneumonia contracted through lying still. No matter how extreme the solution, the risks will always remain.

Avoiding BSE

How do you avoid BSE? By avoiding infected meat. You may choose to stick to recognizable cuts of meat. If you are concerned about beef, turn to other meats. If you are worried about all meat, take advice on vegetarianism. If you feel supermarkets and chain stores dictate to you, don't patronize them. Take control of your decisions. Supermarkets and chain stores exist by cutting costs and trimming corners. Local shops exist on goodwill, and keep in business through trust and word-of-mouth recommendation. Stroll to the butcher and ask advice. Reputable butchers will take meat from a source they know and on whom they rely. They may even raise beef themselves. They will have taken steps to obtain good beef, rather than rejects from the dairy farm. If the sign says 'BSE free' there is every chance it's true.

Since living exposes all of us to risks, a key purpose of government should be to reduce them. When the actions of any system increase personal risk to the individual, then we need to reconsider that system as a matter of urgency. Official reports have often alluded to the need for us to obtain some 'reassurance' about the lack of danger from BSE to human health. It is time the authorities realized that the public do not seek 'reassurance' at all, only truth.

There are, clearly, significant risks to health. They were higher prior to 1990, but the failure to impose safety regulations since then has allowed the hazards to remain greater than they should have been. It is important to set all these risks into context, however. Although life is chancy, even the worst estimates of the danger of beef set the burden into a category comparable with the hazards we regularly accept on the roads, and elsewhere in our daily lives.

The Government's concept of the risk is worth setting out here. The Chief Veterinary Officer, Mr Keith Meldrum, stated in 1990: 'There is no evidence whatever of a risk to human health . . . we have taken measures to deal with BSE.'

Ask him what he thinks of that now, if you can risk it.

16

WHAT SHOULD WE DO?

The story of BSE teaches us many timely lessons. The most important one is that, for all the sense of self-satisfaction it is easy to gain from the science books and television programmes, we still have so much to discover. The infectious agent of the spongy-brain diseases takes us into that fringe area between living and non-living. It is something new. The discovery of the IFDO's in the intestine is another example of this form of agent. We know so little about areas which may turn out to matter so much.

Other lessons we should learn are how ignorant we are about the public perception of risk, and how poorly the great scientific institutes relate their activities to the people whom they influence, and who foot the bills – the public. Science should undergo a process of democratization. We could also pay some attention to the officials who have censored the information, who have prevented research workers from speaking their minds, and who have misled the people.

BSE and AIDS

What of the philosophy of the new diseases? Are BSE, and AIDS, sanctions against unnatural behaviour? It has been claimed that AIDS was nature's way of dealing with homosexuals, which could only be true if measles were nature's answer to the Inuit. In much the same way it has been said that Creutzfeldt-Jakob disease is nature's way of dealing with cannibals. When the Fore people ate their relatives, they developed kuru. When cattle started eating discarded carcases, they developed a similar disease, BSE. Although we must not ignore the extent to which cows naturally digest protozoan (=animal) protein in their normal lives (Chapter 7), there is some common principle here. The short-circuiting of nature's cycles makes it easier for opportunist pathogens to flourish. The characteristic signs of the new spongy-brain disease show that we have a new strain of kuru haunting human society once more.

These terrible brain diseases are spread because of an infectious agent in the diet. Heat sterilization, done properly, would have prevented infection. The lowered standards which followed deregulation allowed a lethal disease to survive in the end products of the feed industry. It is as well we have no current cases of anthrax in Britain. The spores of that dread disease could have withstood the temperatures used to make meat and bone-meal, and it is by good fortune that we have remained free of that. The tolerance of scrapie in sheep has an interesting parallel with *Salmonella* in chicken. Because it has become prevalent, there was a view that it couldn't be eradicated.

This we must change. All such foodstuffs must always be sterilized if there is a chance of starting a reinfection loop from sick animals to healthy stock. This is not a time for penny-pinching. We must make sure these loops do not exist. Waiting until something has gone wrong, and then trying to pick up the pieces, will cost lives. Germs are great opportunists. Sooner or later, they will find a way to exploit any avenue of infection we offer them. Why, there is even an amoeba which lives in unsterilized contact lenses. Heaven knows where that came from, before the contact lens was invented.

Foot-and-Mouth

The response to BSE can be compared with the way we react to other epidemics like foot-and-mouth disease and vesicular disease of swine. Foot-and-mouth is found across much of the globe, but is absent from Australasia, North America and Japan. We no longer have it throughout most of western Europe. Outbreaks are dealt with by immediate slaughter of all cattle in an infected herd and quarantine. Disinfectant blankets are laid on roads near a farm where an outbreak has occurred, so that wheeled vehicles cannot carry a speck of contaminated mud.

Foot-and-mouth is a well-known disease. It was first described, with much accuracy, in 1546. The fact that it was capable of being transmitted by a fluid free of bacteria was determined in 1897, and this gave rise to the fact that some diseases are caused by a 'filterable virus'. It has been studied in the laboratory since the 1920s, and vaccines have been available for years. Foot-and-mouth does not necessarily kill; only 5 per cent of adult animals die, though virtually all become ill. We can gain one possible lesson from the way this virus affects wild animals. They rarely become ill. Buffalo, for example, can catch the virus and show no clinical signs at all. There are doubtless going to be subclinical cases of BSE, but no research has been done to determine their extent.

Vesicular Disease of Swine

This is an extinct epidemic disease that was found in pigs. It makes a fascinating comparison with BSE. The story began in 1932, when there was an outbreak of a disease like foot-and-mouth disease among pigs in California. Every infected animal was slaughtered, the farms quarantined, and the area disinfected. Within months it had been contained. The next outbreak occurred in 1933, and research showed that, though related to foot-and-mouth, this was a new disease. It was given the name *vesicular exanthema of swine* (VES). Regulations were introduced to oblige all those who kept pigs to cook the scraps they were fed. It proved impossible to police, and over the following twenty years outbreaks continued. Up to one-fifth of the entire pig population of southern California was affected, amounting to more than two-and-a-half million animals.

By 1950 the disease was rare. Then, in 1951, a garbage train left San Francisco carrying uncooked pig scraps which were off-loaded in Wyoming. The food went to a single pig-farm. When some of the animals became lame and unwell, the farmer quickly sold them on to farms all over the USA. From 1952 to 1956 outbreaks occurred in forty of the forty-eight states. The laws were tightened. Penalties and policing were increased and many states made it illegal to feed scraps to pigs at all. The last case was in New Jersey in 1956. From that time on there has been no further outbreak, and the disease never escaped from the USA. It is now believed to be extinct, solely because of rigorous action and clear disclosure of the risks.

Comparisons with BSE

There is one glib comparison that can be made. Pigs and cows cost money, so governments act quickly to protect farmers from losses. People are expendable, so a disease of people (like spongy-brain disease) does not cause such a stringent response. That is a political argument, but ignores the facts of the matter. We could take action against foot-and-mouth or VES because the nature of the disease was understood and we knew what we were doing. Spongy-brain disease is new, and does not fit our preconceptions about infections. For instance, it is claimed that a large amount of nerve tissue needs to be ingested before the infection will start. That is unlike any other infection we know. The random decisions can be related in part to this strangeness. On the other hand, it is also true that the Government has often spoken of the need to compensate farmers, and the costs that this will entail. Nothing has been said of compensation to the victims of this killer disease, or of assistance to their families.

The Role of the Media

Official spokesmen have claimed that BSE was a 'media event', and owed much to the current interest in food safety generally. Was the topic a matter of public concern because it was in the media, or was it featured in the media because it was a matter of legitimate public anxiety? The British press are characterized by some of the best science correspondents in the world. Many of them have been laid off by their papers, and now exist as free-lancers, but the quality of their reportage is largely without parallel.

The problems in the media have been caused by the

Government's response. Several of the leading research workers have been ordered not to speak to the press. Some have given off-the-record briefings to journalists at considerable personal risk. British science journalists recognize the pressures, and do not break a confidence. But they often needed a quote, and not merely some additional background. They would be then referred to someone of whom the authorities approved. These spokesmen were always busy, and might suggest that they were telephoned at home in the evening. This is no use to a writer with a deadline to meet, and the scientists never seemed to grasp that essential fact. As a result, many of the journalists ended up telephoning extremist spokesmen whose pronouncements claimed most of the headlines, whilst the truth was never told.

All scientific extremists are recognized by the same criteria:

- They have a record of making doom-laden predictions which have not come true.
- Their predictions lie in the far future, which ensures plenty of repeat bookings by TV programmes.
- Curiously, not unlike many senior politicians, they lack any discernible sense of humour.

Several of these commentators have warned that there will be an epidemic in 2010. Since the original cases of BSE are believed to have occurred about four years after the deregulation of the cattle-feed rendering industry, it would have been scientific to predict that a knock-on infection might itself appear in a similar time-scale. The first cases associated with BSE did indeed occur in 1995, five years after the offal bans were imposed. Why 2010? A sceptic will assume that this was to ensure that participation in programmes might be sought for the next decade and a half.

When Scientists are Silenced

Why do we hear so much from the critics, so much from the Government, yet so little from all the scientists involved? This is the result of policy. We are tolerating a situation where specialists are banned from making public comment, in case the markets might be adversely affected. Such reasoning makes no sense at all. Whenever there have been adverse findings about our daily diet before, we have been told.

In the 1960s, when the epidemiology of cigarette-smoking was first published, nobody dared to suggest that the scientists should keep quiet about their results. There was much in the balance: retail outlets which sell cigarettes would be harmed if demand fell, and manufacturers and importers would suffer too. The revenue from taxation would be disrupted if cigarettes were suddenly unpopular. In spite of these considerations, nobody attempted to interfere with the free expression of information. The spokesmen were open and honest (and surprisingly little happened to the sales of tobacco).

The Legal Dimension

During 1996 a case is being brought through the Scottish courts in which the widow of an Ayrshire smoker who died of lung cancer is suing a major manufacturer for damages. Meanwhile, a group of relatives of victims of the new form of human spongy-brain disease are setting up a case against the British authorities over BSE. The only parallel we have had with BSE is the way that information control was attempted when nuclear disasters happened in the past. The result was immediate – the public was alerted, suspicions were aroused, and people have never had faith in the nuclear industry thereafter.

The public are now aware that infected offal was allowed into our food supply officially until 1989, and has unofficially continued ever since. The infected meat and bone-meal was still on sale for animal feed early in 1996, and now that it has finally been completely outlawed we are still left with those thousands of tons of it spread across the country, with no suggestion as to where it should go. On behalf of the Government, Mr Keith Meldrum MP said in September 1994 that 'we have taken measures to ensure that none of the infected offal from cattle can reach the human food chain'. Many people now take those words with a pinch of salt.

Target for Slaughter

We need to introduce a policy of targeted slaughter as a matter of urgency. The expedient of killing all older cows simply disguises the problem. What we need is cattle of all ages that are not infected with BSE, not cows that are culled before it can become apparent. The great beef herds, most of them free of BSE, the majority fed on grass and home-grown silage, are a priceless part of our farming heritage. The era into which we have been thrust neglects such considerations, but is more closely concerned with the concept of market forces, of basic greed. Once our prime concern was the safety of the public; now people juggle costs and benefits and are sometimes more willing to disguise risks if the chance remains to make money.

Bounty Payments

Clearly, we need to think of a bounty system to encourage farmers and others to report possible outbreaks. Newspaper reports tell how a cattle dealer was fined £30,000 for buying cattle at market and altering their identification so that they seemed to come from BSE-free herds. He was able to collect an extra £100 per beast for the clean bill of health. If a bounty were to be offered, the cash advantage would come for bringing in mad cows, rather than concealing them.

At the heart of the matter is the fact that we have come to tolerate scrapie. The public had not even heard of it until now. We no longer eat mutton, but lamb; and young sheep are slaughtered before the disease has much chance to appear. Every eater of lamb in Europe must be eating a high proportion of meat from animals infected with scrapie. In an ideal world we could eradicate scrapie just as we have eradicated foot-and-mouth disease. It is tempting to think that the idea, for all its theoretical appeal, is impracticable. But it works. Australia and New Zealand are entirely free from scrapie. This is not because they are distant from Europe, and the diseases did not extend that far. On the contrary, it is because of stringent intervention by the authorities. Imported lambs were quarantined, and any found to show the signs of scrapie were immediately slaughtered. Farmers were paid compensation for their losses, and through this strict policy huge areas of the sheep-farming world have been scrapie-free for years.

There are now welcome moves in this direction in Europe. The European Union directive No. 91/68 made scrapie a notifiable disease throughout the Union from 1 January 1993. Typically, in an age of bureaucracy, there is no system of surveillance and little sign of funding to support the scheme. In consequence, nobody knows how widespread the disease really is, and individual animals do not have to be examined at a laboratory even when their herd has been shown to carry the disease. The directive looks good on paper, but means nothing in practice.

We have never considered it practicable to exterminate scrapie. But if it is shown that the scrapie agent has produced BSE – and, in turn, fatal diseases in humans – then we may be faced with a decision to rid our farms of all traces of these infections. We have often heard that, based on the latest evidence, scientists did not believe there is any risk that BSE could be passed to human beings. That is not true. In fact it had never been known whether transmission might take place. There was no evidence it could, but everyone was a little uneasy after the suggestion it might already have passed from sheep to cattle. In Britain we had the lessons of foot-and-mouth disease, from the USA we had the lessons of vesicular exanthema virus of pigs, newly recognized in 1931 yet exterminated, even though it was highly infectious, by 1956. The official response to the new disease of BSE was curious: it was said that the cost of slaughter would be too high. It was also said that, if we were to adopt this approach every time a new disease appeared, there would be no end to the problems we'd face.

Against that was set the likelihood of far greater cost later. That is now coming true. The cost is not just in terms of financial loss to an establishment which supports farming through subsidy, and which lays down the ground rules for how farmers should behave. We now have to face the human cost.

Bringing Science into Government

The most vital new move we need to make is to bring the scientists into the Government. We now have a chief scientific adviser to the Government who is a senior FRS, a dynamic and personable individual, a mathematical master who speaks with authority of concepts in biology. He is Sir Robert May of Oxford University, a breath of fresh air in the corridors of Whitehall. He has acquired much of the official lingo that lurks in Westminster, with mellifluous talk of cost benefits and market efficiency. Clearly he realizes the difficulty faced by any legislative body in a case like this.

In BSE the unknowns are intriguing, and the science remains vague. Admitting this is the way of science, but not of politics. Scientists have been asked to give statements on what to do, but science simply does not know the truth. The Government, meanwhile, wants its aims served by those it funds. Though scientists have begun to understand Parliament, there isn't much to suggest that the politicians have grasped the purpose of science. Neither side has tried to understand the public need for information. Above all, the scientists and politicians still act as though the public do what they are told. In practice, people rarely do what they are advised to do. Several major official reports have advised against saturated fat – so sales of fatty foods go higher by the minute. We have been told to cut back on salt, since when crisps and other salty products increased their sales and are rarely missing from the lunch-box. If there is any single lesson, it is that people often do the opposite of what they have been told. The great anomaly is that the Government advised everyone beef was bound to be safe – had they warned against it, I dare say sales would have doubled in a month.

We must pay close attention to the fate of the infected carcases. Burning them in a pit will not sterilize the remains. BSE is too robust, and higher temperatures are needed to guarantee its destruction. Land-fill burial brings with it the fact that the infective agent is still present in the ground, and could leach elsewhere. One proposal is that the carcases should be minced and disposed of by dumping at sea. Organic matter in the sea is often an excellent idea, for it feeds the tiniest organisms on which all marine life depends. This cannot apply to carcases from animals with BSE. The infective agent is so very resistant that we must be satisfied that it is completely destroyed by incineration, and not spread widely through the marine environment.

Spongy-brain disease remains a mystery. We do not know exactly how it is caused, and have given little thought to a treatment. Even when we speak of its method of transmission we are guessing. The idea that BSE was not likely to be associated with CJD was a guess; the notion that cows were the origin of the new cases of spongy-brain disease in humans is guesswork too. We simply don't know what we are working with, and the story becomes increasingly fascinating as we discover more.

Cost-cutting in the public sector can damage animal welfare and harm public health. If the railways, or water, are privatized then we may run into problems of supply. When we are concerned with health and well-being, epidemics are what await us if the profit motive takes precedence over safety. What we need to do is this:

- We should have health and safety checks at every stage of feed production. This is a multi-million-pound industry, and it must be made aware of its culpability should anything go wrong.
- We should ensure that safety regulations are adhered to in the rearing of animals. Inspection must be thorough, and standards of the highest integrity are crucial.
- Clear labelling is paramount. Consumers need to know what they buy, and farmers must be able to make informed decisions on how they feed their stock.
- The status of the Standing Veterinary Committee in Europe must be maintained, so that the politicians have access to the highest scientific authority.
- Risk assessment must be conducted in an atmosphere without hysteria, and with the full involvement of the public.

- There is an overwhelming need for research into these fundamental problems. Scientific understanding of the mechanisms of these diseases is lacking.
- Competition for grants, and the need to claim attention, causes hyperbole in science. Calm objectivity and reason are often missing.
- Government pronouncements require reappraisal. Open and free discussion of the facts of any scientific topic are vital. Past experience has shown that people are perfectly blasé about the risks that surround us all. They do react violently in situations where they sense that they are not being told the truth.
- Public response to science and understanding of scientific ideas need investigation. Why do people react as they do? How can we encourage them to grasp ideas of science and keep in touch with the fascination of new discovery?
- Legislation must fit the pragmatic requirements of the age. Public safety and the need to protect people from consequences that can kill are vital.
- Treasury planning needs to respond to the demands placed on people by government. If a freely available item of commerce is to be banned, then it is not right that individual concerns should bear the cost. Those who have burdens inflicted on them may recklessly disregard legislation, and too much is now at stake. The proposal for bounty payments to help bring in suspect animals, or for compensation to recover contaminated feed, are examples of where Treasury intervention is important.
- Consultation should be thorough before new rules and regulations are implemented. No farmers were consulted about the proposals to slaughter the entire British herd of cattle aged over thirty months. No experienced vet appeared on the crucial government panels that dealt with the spread of BSE.
- Sudden change is part of the modern world. We must monitor its impact, and study how we can avert problems before they arise.
- If scientific developments impact adversely on the public, they

need recourse to understanding, to support, and perhaps to compensation.

- When science is taken over by politics, truth is soon to go. Science is knowledge: this is our source of insight for the future. It must be untrammelled by political factions and unsullied by short-term expedients.
- There have been discussions on the relaxation of the food hygiene regulations. Any curtailment of bureaucracy is to be welcomed, but there can be no slackening of standards. Food poisoning is increasing, and the BSE epidemic is a lesson in how further outbreaks of novel diseases may occur in the future.

One overwhelming need is a test for spongy-brain disease. One or two simple tests have been claimed in the past, but fell by the wayside. There are hopes that a new test, perhaps of the cerebrospinal fluid around the spine or even of urine, may be announced. On the research front, we must determine how these new discoveries relate to our understanding of diseases and the nature of life.

A Search for a Single Theory

What connections might there be with the other brain diseases which are now widely recognized, but were unknown a few years ago? Alzheimer's is one example. This too is a fatal, degenerative brain disease; as with BSE and CJD, one of the features is a network of fine fibrils which form in the brain. They are not prions, but there could be a common principle behind their formation. Or what of Huntington's disease? This is a genetic condition, in which small fluid-filled spaces start to replace normal brain tissue. Brain degeneration occurs in multiple sclerosis, too, of which we still have little understanding. What of motor neuron disease, in which nerve cells concerned with signalling movement begin to break down? These degenerative afflictions have so much in common. There may well be general principles which unite these dread diseases into a conceptual whole.

It may be that we are on the verge of recognizing common features for a whole new class of human afflictions. We know of viruses, we know about bacteria; we know next to nothing about the causes of these mysterious degenerative diseases. These are our target for tomorrow.

The Prospect for the Future

The spongy-brain diseases are amongst the most fearsome that exist. They are also at the forefront of our understanding. Few brilliant young scientists have come into this field of research in recent years. They don't know what they are missing. The methodical unravelling of the story of scrapie is a scientific saga, and the current work on Creutzfeldt-Jakob disease, and a sudden resurgence of what might be a new strain of kuru in a modern guise, lie at the cutting edge of bioscience. We need new attitudes to tackle them, and new priorities for the future.

The principles for which we must aim are these:

- To banish spongiform diseases. We must tolerate no more massaging of facts. Slaughtering animals before they develop symptoms must never again be considered. BSE must be eradicated, with scrapie next on the list.
- To restore openness in science and medicine. Never before has government interfered so dangerously with the free discussion of results. The hazards of the past – like tobacco, and the problems over saturated fats – have always been fully aired. People make up their own minds.
- To facilitate access to knowledge. Scientists must express their

views openly and directly. The truth about BSE was concealed. In some parts of the world it is unlawful to mention to a sexual partner that an individual has AIDS. If we need laws in such areas, they should ensure that facts are known, and not concealed. Lives hang in the balance through this growing form of secrecy.

- To understand that the creation of knowledge, wisdom and insight are the guiding principles of scientific enquiry. Wealth creation, the guiding light of modern science funding, is irrelevant. Greed is anathema to science.
- To make that great leap, the paradigm shift we need, away from the philosophy of 'cover up and carry on as normal'. If we have public health and well-being to consider, epidemic threats must be eradicated at the outset. The extirpation of disease must apply to BSE; it should then apply to scrapie; it might usefully be extended to *Salmonella* in chickens.
- Feed must be germ-free. We would not tolerate infected food at home, simply because not too many people in the family go sick. We require perfectly wholesome food at all times. So do farm animals. The cost of sterilization is minimal, and germ-free food is easy to obtain.
- No longer must we tolerate the burden of the degenerative diseases. They are a vast spectrum of conditions inflicting suffering on a billion people. Efforts should go into drawing them together in a network of understanding.
- Pure research requires pure funding. Privatization may well work for meteorology or high-energy physics where there is a product in view. But visionary science at the leading edge of thought demands continued funding free from commercial pressures. Pure science in biology is not expensive.

The spongy-brain diseases point up the whole area of degenerative conditions. For medicine to make sense of these is one of our greatest challenges for a new millennium. This is the field for study after genetics, and offers a new revolution in medical knowledge. When government grants for science are targeted at topics like these, young progressive scientists should jump at the chance. A future generation needs their knowledge to help keep suffering to a minimum.

Through greed, expediency, and ignorance of science we have liberated the ancient cannibals' plague in Western society. Insight and integrity should henceforward be our watchword. If we learn the dreadful lessons of the recent past, surely we could turn a lethal legacy into a heritage of hope.

INDEX